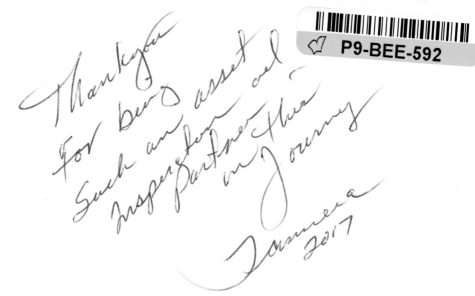

Thank you
For being such an asset and
inspiring partner on this
journey

Tammera
2017

Our Journey with Food

By Tammera J. Karr, PhD

Foreword By James L. Wilson, ND, DC, PhD

Summerland Publishing

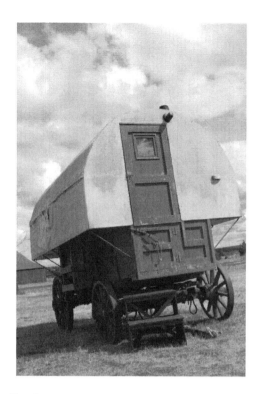

(Photo by Tammera Karr)

The Basque and Irish traveled the remote areas of Oregon, Idaho, Washington and Nevada from the early 20th century to modern times in shepherder's wagons. Today they are pulled behind a four-wheel drive truck and have rubber tires. Soon, they may not exist at all, as this way of life vanishes in the West.

Sheep were taken to high-elevation mountain meadows during the summer and early fall to graze on nutrient-rich grass, lichens and moss. Even today, many of these high meadows are in roadless areas and difficult to reach. A herder would live for months with his dogs out of such wagons.

These herders enjoyed rich, "one-pot meals" and dense, hardy yeast breads, cooked in Dutch ovens or in old coffee cans over a bed of hot coals.

The Basque are world-renowned for their food, which is an important part of their culture.

This Book in any format is not intended to replace recommendations or advice from physicians or other healthcare providers. Rather, it is designed to help you make informed decisions about your health and to cooperate with your healthcare provider in a joint quest for optimal wellness. If you suspect you have a medical problem, we urge you to seek medical attention from a competent healthcare provider.

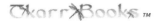 ™

6A Houser Court
Idleyld Park OR 97447 USA

Cover Design JVMedia Design™ 2014
Kitchen life in the 18th century, Skansen, Stockholm, Sweden – Neracc

Photography Credits
Michael W. Karr, Tammera J. Karr, National Archives, Washington, DC
Oregon Historical Society, Portland, Oregon

Proofing Editors *(a thankless job, but ohhh so necessary)*
Carol Rodriguez & Jennifer Furbush

Paperback – ISBN: 978-0-9904864-0-4
IBook - ISBN: 978-0-9904864-1-1
Kindle - ISBN: 978-0-9904864-2-8
Adobe Ebook Reader - ISBN: 978-0-9904864-3-5
Library of Congress Control Number: 2015931833

Author's Note

This book is intended to provide both historical and nutritional information about the foods we eat and have traditionally eaten as a society. It includes many direct quotes from original case studies, scientific journals and other reputable sources. All of the research sources are located in the footnotes. Supplementing the text are several historical photographs culled from archives, libraries and museums. I hope you enjoy the Journey.

Reviews

Tammera writes likes she talks. Weaving history into today's relevant awareness is Tam's special knack. She has a robust and insatiable appetite in her personal quest for answering questions that drive her. I say thank you for distilling the complexities of food and diet into usefulness! Thank you for sharing the treasures that you have gathered over the years with all of us!
Lorrie Amitrano, FNP, AHN, CNP

Tammera Karr's *Our Journey With Food* is absolutely jam-packed with relevant and important information about nutrition and real health (not just the absence of disease). It also contains loads of fun facts about our sources of nourishment. Did you know that the thickness of onion skins have been used to predict the severity of the oncoming winter? Of course Tammera would know that, she's the most down-to-earth, *Farmer's Almanac*, foodie-nutritionist, around!

Thanks Tam for creating this awesome resource that will not only help save lives with the well-researched information it contains, but will provide great fodder for interesting discussion around many a dinner table.
Susan Barendregt, Functional Nutritionist

Here we are at the top of the food chain and we're more confused about what to eat than ever before. In *Our Journey With Food*, Tammera Karr provides us with a glimpse into the past and explains how and why we've lost our connection with healthy food. This book is not only a fascinating and fresh look at past culinary traditions, it's also a wake-up call to get back to the basics — unprocessed, healthful, wholesome foods.

Melissa McLean Jory, MNT
Author of The Gluten-Free Edge

Tammera Karr's *Our Journey with Food* is a must-read. Tammera has the uncanny ability to take complicated physiology, vitamins, minerals, statistics, and the confusion over what to eat, and break it down into easy-to-understand-and-digest chunks. A resource you will refer back to over and over.

Americans are some of the unhealthiest citizenry in the world. How did this happen? Why did this happen? Tammera answers these questions and so many more as she takes you through a journey through the history of our food. Full of facts and interesting statistics that will blow your mind.

Learn which foods are best for the prevention of cancer, fatigue, diabetes, and hormonal health challenges; the why is backed with the latest research, which now supports what holistic nutrition practitioners have always known.

Consume chocolate, eggs including the yolks, meat and alcohol in confidence once again while taking in all the great tips and anecdotes. Yes, you heard me right! What nutritionist covers alcohol? Learn the health effects and benefits connected to alcohol and how to make wassail! Wow! this is one powerhouse, fact-packed book.

Karen Langston CNCP, CN, LM, SIT
Holistic Nutritionist specializing in digestive health
KarenLangston.com

Our Journey with Food is an honest and enlightening look at the healthful aspects of our food. Tammera presents a wealth of information about how food impacts our physical health, making this a must-have resource for everyone.

Rebekah Fedrowitz, MHN, BCHN

What Calls Me

My cells carry the memories of my ancestors—
they call out to be remembered and to remind.

My blood surges with the song of family—
the past whispers, the present sings, and the future dances on the fringes of the
mind.

I sing out what I have learned, of remembrance and tell the story of our history, of
tradition, family and responsibility.

My cells carry the memory of our ancestors,
our past, present and our hope in times yet to come.

by Tammera J. Karr

Dedication

This and so much more I owe to my best friend, soul mate and love, Michael. To my son Brendan who has heard it all, and like his dad subject to being a guinea pig mostly with good grace. To Matthew, childhood and adult co-conspirator, I love you. For my sister Donna, who loved me more than I knew, and who became a memory all too soon. And to my mother-in-law Libby who trusted me to the end.

In the healthcare world, having mentors has been a must. These individuals are family nurse practitioners, acupuncturists, chiropractors, doctors of osteopathic medicine, naturopaths, nutritionists, compounding pharmacists, educators, researchers and authors. With their help I have learned about patient care, follow-up, cooperation, expectations, flexibility and value.

With deep thanks to Mary, Lorrie, Susan, Darryl, Marty and Paul.

Special thanks to the crew at JVMedia who developed cover designs, marketing tools and more. To the editors of the *Roseburg Beacon*, David and Marilyn, who have given me the opportunity to write. And to Jennifer who put in as many hours proofing as I did writing.

To all the clients I have seen over the years; thank you for sharing a part of your life with me.

This book has been made possible by the generous donations of:

Matthew M. Davies

Michael W. Karr

Jean Caskey

Dr. Darryl B. George

Karen Gibbons

Anonymous Angel

Mary L. Hagood

Mr. & Mrs. Lee Tyler

Anonymous Angel

Ruth Kummrow

Lorrie Amitrano

Shirley & Clyde Pyle

Jacque Everden

M. A. Hansen

Table of Contents

We live in an age in which doctors and scientists are specializing more and more, building their reputations and careers around being experts in ever-narrowing areas of expertise. This has allowed us to make significant advances in medicine and science, but has also left us drowning in a tsunami of often conflicting bits of information that are too overwhelming and confusing to be useful in our daily lives. What is lacking but greatly needed are generalists who can meaningfully integrate all the bits of information generated by specialists, and impart that understanding in a practical way to the rest of us. A very important area desperately in need of unbiased, knowledgeable generalists is the connection between food, nutrition and health because it plays such a central role in our ability to lead full and healthy lives.

I believe Dr. Karr is one of these much needed but rare generalists with no vested interest or ulterior motive except to integrate and synthesize information in a way that both makes sense and is useful. In *Our Journey with Food*, Dr. Karr has provided a sourcebook integrating extensive scientific, historical and traditional information from the fields of food, nutrition and health. She writes from the perspective of one who loves and understands the subject based on her academic training, clinical expertise and hands-on experience living in the wilds of Oregon.

With a grassroots style that is almost folksy at times, she tells it like it is, as a person who has real experience with food—growing, storing, cooking and studying it—and also as a professional with academic knowledge and a clear grasp of practical applicability. This is an unusual book combining many scientific facts, anecdotes, folk tales, history and photos, as well as political issues and fallacies around food and specific nutrients. She does a nice job of debunking the cholesterol and fat myths, and emphasizes the devastating effects of white sugar and flour, while revealing the influences of agribusiness and politics on our daily food intake without being too sinister or fatalistic.

So this book is indeed a "Journey with Food" that also provides a succinct rundown on each of the major vitamins and minerals and their roles in health, plus the medicinal uses of some foods. It makes for entertaining reading!

When so much of the United States' gross domestic product (GDP) depends upon sickness, you know that overall health in this country is not nearly as good as we would like to believe. One significant reason for this is that many people no longer recognize good food when they see or taste it, let alone know how to grow, store and cook it. Their taste buds have become so distorted with the excess sugar and artificial sweeteners and flavors present in much of the typical North American diet that if they shift to a diet of natural foods, it takes them approximately six weeks to be able to fully taste the natural flavors. Food has been defined and redefined to fit so many political and economic purposes, but for me the definition of food is simple: Real food is that which comes from or runs around on the ground, or lives in the water. In short, if it does not look like it was once alive it probably is not real food.

Most of you familiar with my writing know that stress and its effects on endocrine function and the overall balance of the body (homeostasis) is a central topic of my work. I can attest from decades of clinical and research experience that without making real food the major component of daily consumption, it is almost impossible to recover from stress, adrenal fatigue, or other forms of debilitation and illness. It is also true that without the basic ingredient of good food, it is very difficult to be and remain healthy and withstand the stresses of life. Food is the raw material that becomes the body. Just as in building a house, substandard raw materials cannot produce a house that will withstand the storms of life.

Too many people drive themselves with caffeine and quick energy concoctions instead of obtaining real energy from good quality foods. Most cannot even imagine functioning properly without their caffeine and sugar fixes. Combine this with the high consumption of over-the-counter, prescription and street drugs and it is not surprising that a large portion of the population no longer knows what it is like to wake up feeling refreshed, healthy and eager to meet the day. We are on a runaway train careening from fast food restaurants to doctor's offices, while accepting these diminished or debilitated states of life as normal. Because we have forgotten or never knew we could be healthy by eating real food and leading less stressful lives, we continue to exist in desensitized overloaded states, just striving to remain functional. This is now so common we do not even recognize how unusual it is to live life unencumbered by sickness, partial disability or degeneration before our time. We must change!

So thank you, Dr. Karr, for writing this book! It is a place where people can find practical guidance on how to incorporate real food as the major portion of their daily diet, as well as answers that lead the way back to health. With the shift in healthcare currently taking place in the U.S., there will be an ever greater divide between the people who know how to live a healthy lifestyle and take care of themselves, and those who depend on the medical system for their "health" (i.e. sick) care. Over time the former will fare much better. We would all greatly benefit from having more generalists like Dr. Karr who have lived their subjects as she has lived food, nutrition and health.

James L. Wilson, DC, ND, PhD, author of
Adrenal Fatigue: The 21st Century Stress Syndrome

My journey into the world of natural health began in the late 1970s when a great aunt gave my mother a copy of the book *Back to Eden* by Jethro Klause. It wasn't long before the book caught my attention and my newfound passion was inspired. Years later, I went from being a "dabbler" to a serious student of nutrition.

In 1996, I became a nutraceutical representative. This came about, not because of a drive for a home-based business, but because my best friend and husband was daily enduring chronic pain due to a motorcycle accident. There were more days than I care to remember when he was unable to sit upright or play with his toddler son due to the pain from damaged discs in his back and severe, nerve-pinching muscle spasms.

We took some herbal supplements and ate reasonably well, but it wasn't until my husband tried a liquid mineral supplement from humus plant sources that pain relief occurred. That single event propelled me to learn more about nutrition and how it might help my family. With the encouragement of friends and a chiropractor, I started distance schooling in the field of holistic nutrition. I don't know if it was because I had already been working with nutritional products or if I was just a natural, but before I knew it I had completed my bachelor's of science degree and signed on for the master's and the doctorate of holistic nutrition programs.

In 2002, I was offered an opportunity to work with a small alternative medical group in rural Southern Oregon. Everything I thought I knew quickly went out of the window as I was introduced to clients who were dealing with such issues as having more titanium in their backs than bone, failed gastric bypasses, migraines, glaucoma, rheumatoid arthritis, diabetes 1 and 2, hepatitis C, thyroid and endocrine system illnesses, PTSD, depression, bipolar disorder, drug addiction and cancer. School was now truly in session, and these folks were desperate for help.

In time I was introduced to national accreditation bodies and have since dedicated time to serving on their various boards. I am very proud of the work being done by the National Association of Nutrition Professionals and the American Association of Integrative Medicine to further the profession of holistic nutritionists, integrated, culturally traditional medicine, and natural health and dietary modalities. The students graduating from schools like the Wellspring School of Healing Arts are a joy to mentor and give me confidence in the work I and many others are doing to build a brighter future for natural health practitioners.

Clients' symptoms vary from brain fog, leg cramps and digestive complaints to more serious conditions such as Parkinson's disease, MS, cancer and the rare Pick's Disease (rapid deterioration of the brain's frontal lobe). So many of these degenerative and chronic illnesses could have been prevented with real food and optimized nutrition.

One of the topics I have chosen to write about involves alcoholic drinks. I know this can be a controversial subject for nutritionists to write about, but the fact remains that I have told clients countless times to eliminate alcohol for their blood sugar levels, waistline and health, but they rarely do. I found myself wondering about all the reasons why. There are the obvious ones about deficiency cribbing, brain chemistry, self-medication, addiction and diabetic sugar cravings. However, I thought there had to be more to this question and began looking into the history of spirits, beer and wine and how they affect our health and our innate desire to imbibe. The story is long and may be surprising.

Over time, I have developed a theory that "our cells carry the memories of our ancestors." All of us are suffering from progressive generational malnutrition. Each successive generation that digresses further from our ancestral and "real" foods former diet suffers more genetic and nutritional imbalances and more chronic, life-shortening illnesses. Fortunately, the new field of nutrigenomics is validating the superiority of real foods over those synthesized by man.

Every year, science opens more doors of understanding into the wisdom and knowledge of our ancestors. Ancient man did not need a microscope or mass-spectrometer to determine what foods and herbs to eat, they learned from experience and observation. Throughout time, this knowledge was passed forward until "modern" medicine and technology overshadowed common sense and tradition.

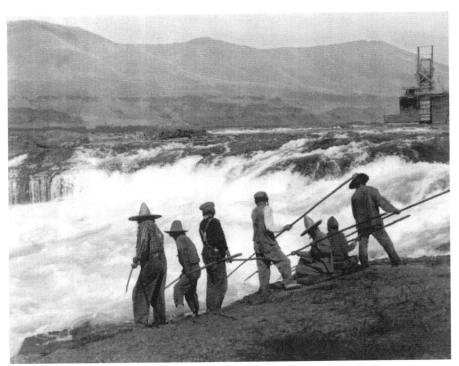

Native Americans fishing at Celilo Falls on the Columbia River, 1950s. Photo by Benjamin Gifford – OHS Image BB001038. The roughly horseshoe-shaped falls 14 miles upstream from present-day The Dalles, Oregon, were one of two important Native American fishing and trading places on the Columbia River. Celilo Falls disappeared under the water behind The Dalles Dam in 1957. Bonneville Power Agency operates and maintains about three-fourths of the high-voltage transmission in its service territory which includes Idaho, Oregon, Washington, western Montana and small parts of eastern Montana, California, Nevada, Utah and Wyoming.

The following pages will detail some of the information from patient studies, clinical research and practical application garnered over my years of private practice in the fields of holistic nutrition and integrative medicine.

Food is very much a part of our history and our health. Enjoy the journey.

Tammera

In 1973 Reay Tannahill wrote a book that today is still considered one of the most comprehensive works on food history. The aptly titled *Food in History* covers man's selections of foods from prehistoric to the modern age. At last, here was a book that spoke to my love of history as well as food. From here I began collecting works such as *Near a Thousand Tables: A History of Food* by Felipe Fernandez-Armesto, *Empires of Food* by Evan D.G. Fraser, and similar historical tomes. One day I came across *The Taste of War* by Lizzie Collingham and *Botany of Desire* by Michael Pollan and my vision changed from past to present.

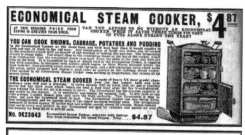

Toledo "Fireless" Steam Cooker

This stove top steam cooker was manufactured by the Toledo Cooker company of Toledo, Ohio. Near the turn of the 20th century the cookers were very popular. This is a listing in the 1908 Sears Catalog for the Toledo Cooker.

Catalogue advertisement provided by the Bowman Museum Prineville, Oregon

As I read, I saw our travels taking us from continent to country to state. As I learned about our ancestors' quest for new foods, farm land, commercial enterprise and new methods of food preservation, a realization dawned. I began to see how much food has shaped our heritage and history on this continent. Nourishment, sustenance, food; no matter what you call it, it has been sought out by explorers long before the works of Frank N. Meyer and P.H. Dorsett coined the term "agricultural explorers" in the late 1800s. We are dirt farmers, ranchers, truck drivers, teachers, doctors and stockbrokers, all living our lives because of the one ingredient that is the foundation of life—food.

Most of the world sees food as a healer as well as a source of primal nourishment. Unfortunately, many of us who live in the contemporary United States have forgotten about the role of food as healer and cultural treasure. We want it fast, easy, with no muss or fuss; we want the high, the sweet, the satisfaction. And so we have developed into a country with a chronically ill population, confused by what food is good for us and what is not (if we can even call these new-fangled processed products "food").

In the 1950s most households had televisions, which brought about the advent of "TV dinners" and mindless eating in front of the screen. Food product development and marketing became an exciting, fast-growing field.

"While the frozen turkeys rode the rails, Gerry Thomas, a shrewd Swanson & Sons salesman, traveled from his company's base in Nebraska to the kitchens of Pan American Airways in Pittsburgh. At the time, Pan Am was testing single-compartment foil trays used to serve warm in-flight meals to passengers. Thomas 'borrowed' one of the trays (conveniently slipping it into his coat pocket) and spent his return trip drawing up plans for a three-compartment version that would ensure that peas and gravy would never touch each other."[1]

CorningWare, the white cookware decorated with blue cornflowers, has been a fixture at family gatherings and potlucks for decades.

"S. Donald Stookey is credited with creating a synthetic ceramic glass in the 1950s that led to the famous cookware brand. Stookey discovered glass ceramics in 1952—the fortuitous outcome of an experiment gone wrong."

The durable cookware, able to withstand extreme temperatures, became one of the housewife's best kitchen finds of the 1950s-1970s. "CorningWare was the first cookware of the modern age to go from freezer to oven to table. Later, CorningWare was used in microwave ovens and on cooktops."[2, 3]

Tupperware, invented by Earl Tupper, began appearing in every home in America in the 1950s as well.

"A dynamic single mom with a knack for marketing took a plastic container invented in 1946 from obscurity to essential kitchen staple." This was the dawn of a new age of plastic containers and storage bags. Americans had not yet heard of the xenobiotic dangers they presented to our endocrine systems.[4, 5]

Before the microwave oven became a fixture in homes, circa 1960, *The I Hate to Cook Book* was impacting millions of kitchens in the United States and abroad. Peg Bracken's cookbook quickly became a staple of suburban homes. She believed that ingredients should be cheap, common and above all convenient, ideally frozen or tinned. Canned soups were a main ingredient in her recipes. So were crushed cornflakes, powdered onion soup mix and Spam. Alcohol had its place as well,

[1] http://www.gourmet.com/food/gourmetlive/2011/101911/the-history-of-the-tv-dinner
[2] http://www.npr.org/blogs/thetwo-way/2014/11/07/362226389/scientist-who-invented-corningware-glass-dies-at-99
[3] http://www.classickitchensandmore.com/page_3.html
[4] http://www.pbs.org/wgbh/americanexperience/films/tupperware/player/
[5] http://stri.si.edu/english/research/facilities/library/index.php

though in many cases Bracken's instructions called for it to bypass the cooking process entirely and proceed straight down the cook's throat.[6]

Bracken's book opened the doors of home kitchens to mega-food manufacturers; Rice-a-Roni, American Cheese and Hamburger Helper are just some of the processed foods, still prevalent in stores and homes today, that were used for convenience cooking by low-income and working families. Most people have no idea about the cooking revolutions that took place in 1960s kitchens, the opposing views of Julia Child and Adelle Davis, and the results that Bracken's quick-fix recipes had on Americans' health.

In 1955, "the Tappan Stove Company, under a licensing agreement with Raytheon, brought the first consumer microwave ovens to the U.S. market with a price tag of $1,300. In 1965, Raytheon acquired Amana Refrigerators, Inc., and in 1967, it introduced to the U.S. market the first 'countertop' model of microwave ovens (it sold for $495 retail and was smaller, safer and more reliable than previous models). By 1986, 25 percent of U.S. households owned a microwave oven, up from less than one percent in 1971." (Microwave Oven Regression Model, U.S. Bureau of Labor Statistics). [7, 8]

During this time period, science and technology seemed to promise an ever more convenient, beautiful future for the denizens of post-war America. Each product was better, faster and sleeker than the last.

Many of our contemporary opinions about food can be traced to the beginnings of the Clean Food movement of the 1960s[9] and "the diet age", which really took off in the 1970s. The Age of Aquarius introduced us to "the grapefruit diet" (revived from the 1950s), and, in the mid-1970s, Elvis Presley popularized the "Sleeping Beauty Diet" in which he was heavily sedated for several days, hoping to wake up thinner. Actress Twiggy introduced us to vegetarianism, which, though seen as faddish at the time, is now still a popular lifestyle choice.

Low-calorie plans were promoted by actress Farah Fawcett (simultaneously, and perhaps not coincidentally, a startling increase in anorexia began during the 1970s, jeopardizing many young women's lives). Macrobiotic and Ayurvedic approaches were also popular. These protocols were undoubtedly far healthier than the snazzy new "diet" and weight-loss foods appearing on grocery store shelves that resembled desserts, such as the low- fat "chocolate" chews and drinks.

---

[6] http://www.nytimes.com/2007/10/23/arts/23bracken.html?_r=0
[7] http://www.bls.gov/cpi/cpimwo.htm
[8] http://www.bls.gov/cpi/cpimwo.htm_truncated
[9] The Complete Idiots Guide to Clean Eating 2009, Diane Welland, MS, RD

Low-fat diets were all the rage in the 1980s and supermodels like Christie Brinkley produced workout videos to thin us down. This misguided approach ignored our bodies' need for a vital nutrient found in real unprocessed food: fats.

In the 1990s, the work done by Dr. Barry Sears, Gean and Joyce Daoust, Dr. Robert Atkins[10] and Ann Louise Gittleman, PhD, illustrated the need for a balance between the macronutrients of protein, fat and carbohydrates. In this decade, we were introduced to the Mediterranean Diet, the Atkins Plan™, 40-30-30, the Perricone Prescription Diet™ and the pH Diet. Medical professionals began getting involved in the nutrition arena; perhaps this was due to a savvy business sense, or perhaps it was due to their frustration at seeing their patients' health failing on the conventional diets of the day.

Now science has catapulted us into nutrigenomics, DNA/RNA activators, and a far better understanding of bio-individuality, the idea of tailoring different lifestyle choices to different individuals. We are learning about the inherent nutritional superiority of real whole foods over processed and refined ingredients (much to the horror of the commercial food industry and political lobbyists).

Newfound understanding of the genes involved in taste perception and food preferences can lead to personalized nutrition plans, which can be effective not just in terms of weight loss but in preventing diseases like cancer, depression and hypertension.

"The ability to devise diets based on individual genetic profiles can lead to significantly better results—for example, a weight loss 33% greater than with a control group who had a similar calorie count but a non-personalized diet plan," researchers from the European Society of Human Genetics (ESHG) say.[11]

Farming has changed dramatically since the 1970s. A 2014 NPR feature highlighted a few of the changes: "According to the latest census of American agriculture, released in 2014, there are two million farms in America.[12] But just four percent of those farms account for two-thirds of all agricultural production."[13]

---

[10] http://www.shape.com/blogs/weight-loss-coach/dieting-through-decades-what-weve-learned-fads
[11] European Society of Human Genetics (ESHG). "Revolutionizing diets, improving health with discovery of new genes involved in food preferences." ScienceDaily. ScienceDaily, 1 June 2014. <www.sciencedaily.com/releases/2014/06/140601201954.htm>.
[12] http://www.agcensus.usda.gov/
[13] http://www.npr.org/blogs/thesalt/2014/06/16/321705130/in-the-making-of-megafarms-a-few-winners-and-many-losers?sc=ipad&f=1001

According to a National Geographic article, "Large corn and soy farms in the midwest may cover up to 16,000 acres, which equates to 25 square miles of farmland." *(In The Making Of Megafarms, A Mixture Of Pride And Pain, June 16, 2014)* At one time, dozens of smaller farms covered the same area of land, and tens of families were supported by their agrarian lifestyle. Today, two men with just seven full-time employees are doing the work that hundreds did just a few decades ago. Those seven or ten workers plant the seeds, spread the fertilizer and keep the irrigation water flowing. The farm managers spend as much time inside monitoring their crops on computers as they once did out in the field, deliberating what seeds to buy, when to plant and when to sell their harvest.

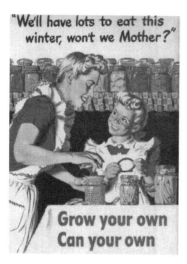

Illustration from the National Archives Washington, D.C.

Currently there seems to be a slight rebounding of small, family farms as more people realize the health benefits of locally produced food. A niche market for homespun goods is reappearing in American culture, similar to what was seen during the Great Depression and World War II. Farmers' markets are cropping up from coast to coast, and in some areas such as Washington, D.C., activists are introducing the public to healthy foods via mobile farm market vans. People are also learning how to prepare and preserve their homegrown produce, and canning, fermenting and other food preservation methods are making a comeback in American kitchens.

The implementation of the Pure Food and Drug Act of 1906 made it illegal to sell products doctored with toxic chemicals.[14] John McMonigle and Charles Wille served one year in Leavenworth Prison, in 1886 and 1915, respectively, for the crime of selling margarine, or oleo, recorded as "crimes against butter".[15] In today's world there are dozens of margarine products for consumers to buy, yet at the turn of the 20th century it was considered a health hazard.

---

[14] What's Cooking Uncle Sam? Records from the National Archives pg. 28
[15] What's Cooking Uncle Sam? Records from the National Archives pg. 13

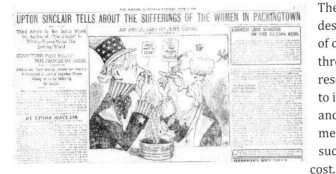

Illustration From the National Archives, Washington, D.C.

The Hatch Act of 1887 was designed to "sow the seeds of creativity in every state" through land grants and research stations dedicated to improving agricultural and food production methods. In a way, it was a success—but not without a cost.

In terms of productivity and efficiency, a collective increase in the use of chemical fertilizers, herbicides and pesticides makes perfect sense. Subsequent bills passed in the 1930s helped regulate supply and demand.[16] This race for bigger, faster and better has moved beyond the application of chemicals and into the realm of altering the genetic code of living organisms. Multi-billion dollar agribusinesses such as Monsanto® and Cargill® are splicing dog DNA into corn and cholera into potatoes.

The idea that the scientist has more to offer us than the farmer has led us to inventions such as artificial sweeteners (which can affect cognition and harm pancreatic function), processed fats plugging our arteries and Senomyx™[17] (aborted fetal tissue) in soda pop.[18]

Too bad that the Pure Food and Drug Act of 1906[19, 20] has been buried in a quicksand of time, politics and "progress". Undoubtedly, the writers of that bill would balk at the amount of chemicals, many with little to no safety data, that are being introduced into our food supply. I suspect that lawmakers of the day would have locked Monsanto and its cohorts up into Leavenworth and thrown away the key.

While large corporate mega-giants are without a doubt "doing what it takes" to make billions, consumer responsibility also plays a role in deciding what's found on our grocery store shelves.

The Internet has made it possible for activists and average citizens critical of GMOs and industrial-chemical farming methods to rally millions of supporters to their

---

[16] Agricultural Adjustment Act 1933
[17] http://en.wikipedia.org/wiki/Senomyx
[18] http://articles.mercola.com/sites/articles/archive/2013/03/17/senomyx-flavor-enhancers.aspx
[19] http://www.loc.gov/rr/news/topics/purefood.html
[20] http://www.encyclopedia.com/topic/Food_and_Drug_Act_of_1906.aspx

cause. It has also proved a fertile field for frauds and charlatans hawking the next "miracle" cure or diet.

Keep in mind that efforts to combat obesity can be a threat to businesses that produce and sell food: If people eat less, profits will decline. The food industry can't appear to be nonresponsive to what has been termed a public health crisis, so it employs several tactics to maintain legitimacy and position itself as "part of the solution" while also protecting profits. Food companies tend to frame obesity as solely the consequence of the choices people are making rather than the choices they are being offered, say researchers at George Washington University.[21]

Buzzwords like "antioxidant", "gluten-free" and "whole grain" deceive consumers into thinking food products are healthier than they actually are, according to a new research study. That "false sense of health" as well as a failure to understand the information presented in nutrition facts panels may be contributing to the obesity epidemic in the United States, say researchers at the University of Houston.[22]

---

[21] George Washington University. "Is the food industry really concerned with obesity? If people eat less, profits will decline." ScienceDaily. ScienceDaily, 2 June 2014. <www.sciencedaily.com/releases/2014/06/140602150703.htm>.
[22] University of Houston. "How food marketing creates false sense of health." ScienceDaily. ScienceDaily, 13 June 2014. <www.sciencedaily.com/releases/2014/06/140613130717.htm>.

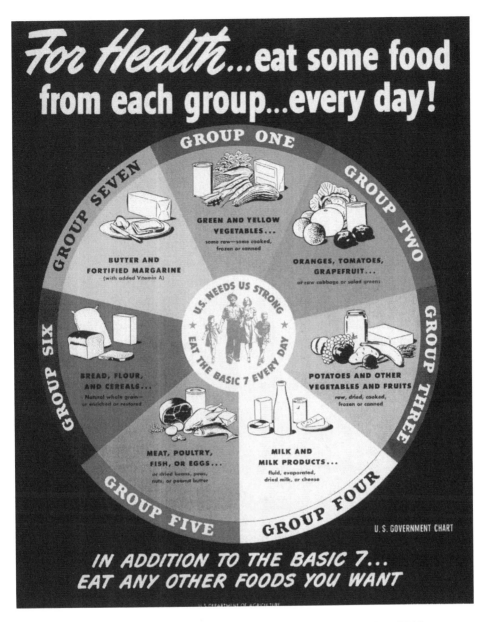

Second Food Recommendation Chart to be published by the USDA in 1945; precursor to today's food guides. *(National Archives Washington, D.C.)*

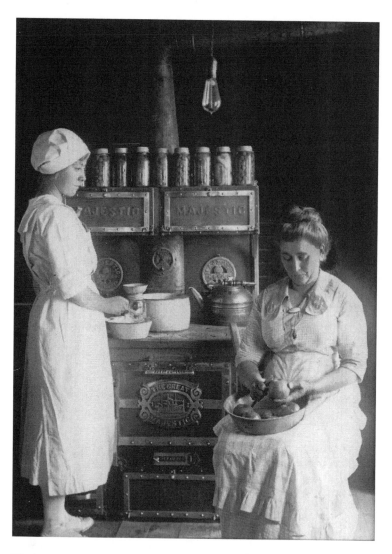

Kitchen in an upscale home in Oregon City, Oregon, circa 1900. Due to Oregon Falls on the Willamette River and the hydroelectric plant established in the 1800s, Oregon City was the first area to transmit commercial electricity in the United States (in 1889, to Portland, Oregon). Oregon City was established in 1842 by Dr. John McLoughlin, the "Father of the Oregon Territory" *(Historic Photograph print by Alex Blendl).*

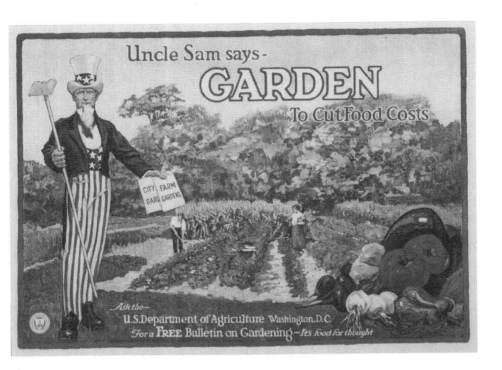

Victory Gardens were an important part of the war effort in 1917. Similarly, during the Great Depression and circa 1942, every household that could planted a garden to keep food on the table. The home farm extension program provided free seeds to families who couldn't buy them. *(National Archives, Washington, D.C.)*

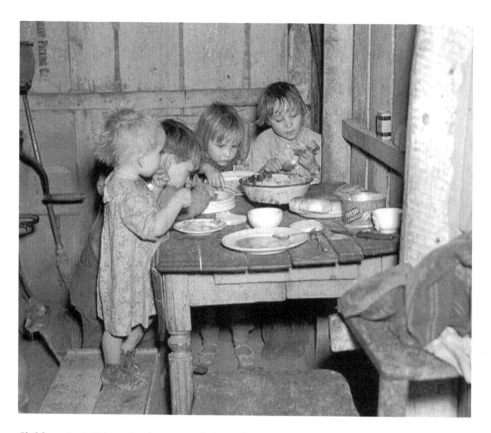

Children in 1930 eating homemade bread, boiled turnips and cabbage. Back then, all produce was "organic" by default, and food was grown locally by the family or local farmers.

In the 1930s, the Civilian Conservation Corps (CCC) built roads, trails and buildings all over the nation. This civilian army had to be fed. But the food that fueled this labor-intensive work was not today's institutional food. Companies like Kellogg's provided the CCC with tin boxes filled with recipes and menus for every day of the week.

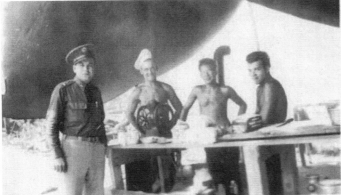

Tennessee CCC menu February 3rd, 1937[23]

Breakfast: Stewed Peaches - Boiled Rice - Fresh Milk - Hot Biscuits - Fried Bacon - Scrambled Eggs - Coffee

Lunch: Macaroni & Cheese - Cold Tomatoes - Lima Beans - Fried Cabbage-Dried Peach Cobbler - Coffee

Supper: Fried Beef Steak - Brown Gravy - Fried Eggplant - Green Beans - Cream Cauliflower - Butter & Jam with Bread

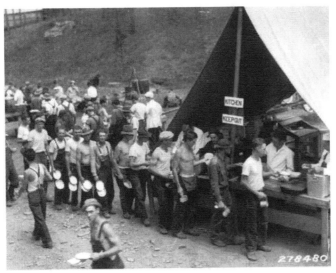

---

[23] "Favorite Recipes of the United States Conservation Corps 1933-1942" (Spiral-bound)

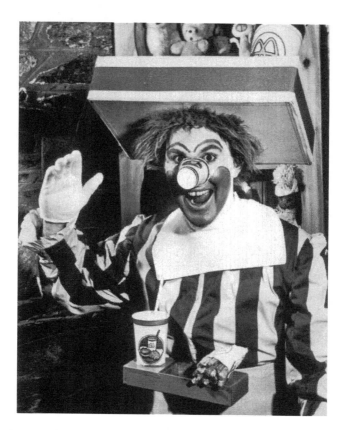

In 1940, brothers Richard and Maurice McDonald opened their first restaurant in San Bernardino, California.[24] Fast food chain restaurants like McDonald's started becoming prevalent in the 1960s. One of the first Ronald McDonald clown mascots was designed in 1963. Ray Kroc later took the franchise global; today, there are more than 35,000 locations worldwide. A 2013 Ad Age compilation of the 25 largest U.S. advertisers ranked McDonald's as the fourth largest advertiser, spending $957,000,000 on advertisements in 2012. The fast food industry is the most heavily advertised sector of the U.S. economy, spending over 4.6 billion dollars in 2012.[25,26]

[24] TIME Dec 29, 2014: 2015 The Year Ahead, pg 112
[25] Fast Food Marketing Ranking Tables 2012-2013. Yale. Retrieved January 25, 2014
[26] Meet America's 25 biggest advertisers. AdAge. Retrieved July 8, 2013

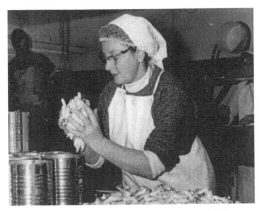

OHS Image bb012650 – Lucille Stewart packs first crabs to come into Yaquina Bay. December 5, 1963. Point Adams Packing Co. Newport, Oregon

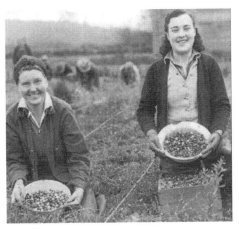

OHS Image bb012654– November 10, 1940. Mrs. Ella Worthington (left), champion cranberry picker of the penninsula in Pacific County, Washington, and Mrs. Joe Weisner display measures of cranberries. Mrs. Worthington averages 20 measures a day.

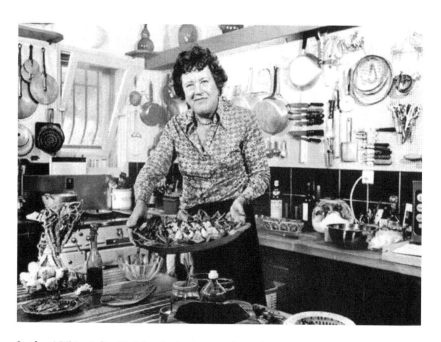

In the 1950s, Julia Child splashed onto the culinary scene and radically changed how American women entertained and cooked. In 1963, this remarkable lady took over TV sets with the first of many cooking shows. Julia Child won a Primetime Emmy® Award for "Achievement in Educational Television" for *The French Chef*, in 1966, becoming the first educational television personality to receive an Emmy in open competition. Her energetic and free spirit laid the foundations for today's cooking programs, networks, websites, bloggers and authors.

Photo American History Museum Smithsonian, Washington D.C.

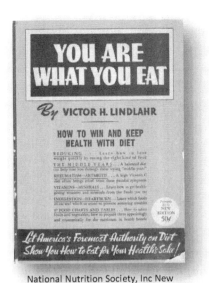

National Nutrition Society, Inc New York 1942

Allopathic medicine treats symptoms with targeted medications. However, complications from side effects can result in more medications being prescribed, and polypharmacy is the outcome. One common but rarely addressed side effect is nutritional deficiencies, which can lead to cascading symptomology and degeneration.

Many patients are under the impression that their healthcare providers have training in nutrition and are keeping up with current research. More often than not, this is not the case. Patients may become the victims of "practice" or "routine", often times due to physicians being driven by insurance and government regulations.

This combined with the current state of food production[27] has resulted in a country with some of the unhealthiest citizenry in the world. Unfortunately, many clients who seek care for chronic pain management are so consumed with the pain and stress of chronic illness that the last thing on their minds is healthy eating. Instead of considering what their dietary choices may be doing to their mind and body, they just want a pill to make the pain stop as quickly as possible.

Whenever someone recounts a miraculous improvement after the use of a new supplement, I immediately know that individual has significant nutritional issues and, in a matter of time, their dramatic results will fade. The basic physiological reasons are, as cell receptor sites open and receive long lost or insufficient nutrients, they at first respond in an over-excited manner (which can result in sudden, dramatic improvements in well-being). As time passes, generally after 90 to 180 days, the receptor sites have been "reset" and moderate their response.

Some individuals will experience positive results for longer periods of time depending on the nutrient they are taking (this is generally the case for ionic minerals and B vitamins).

---

[27] (Howell, 1985)

Psychologically, four other factors play into the effectiveness of natural health protocols and the overall outcome:

1. *Complacency.* As individuals begin to feel better, or their symptoms resolve, they become less compliant or stop the nutritional program they are on, whether it is a liquid supplement, intravenous therapy or a tailored nutrient delivery program.
2. *Carelessness.* The clients forget why they are taking the nutraceuticals, stretching or walking every day. I have also seen clients repeatedly sabotage their success by second guessing their natural health practitioner and adding more supplements from retailers.
3. *Confusion.* When relaying information to clients it is common for them to have lost the information before they have made it across the parking lot. Recommendations need to be in a form that clients can read and understand. A hand-scrawled note often will result in noncompliance.
4. *Cost.* For whatever reason, individuals can justify the purchase of fake fingernails, beer, alcohol, video games, cigarettes, pet care and junk food but they fail to see the cost-benefits and paramount importance of cleaning up their diet and using quality nutraceuticals.

What is Holistic Nutrition?

❖ Holistic Nutrition looks at the total person and their unique biochemical responses to their environment, dietary intake, supplements and lifestyle.

❖ Holistic Nutritionists believe food is our most important medicine, and should be addressed first in the healing process.

❖ Holistic Nutritionists interface with healthcare practitioners, aiding in addressing chronic health challenges that respond to changes in real food and supplement protocols along with addressing allergens, deficiencies and imbalances.

❖ Holistic Nutrition honors dietary needs based on ethnicity, religious and philosophical beliefs; incorporates appropriate holistic health modalities; and promotes wellness of the mind, body and spirit.

In order to live we must eat. But what we eat and why, and the cumulative effects on the body systems, can create a complex story. Let's begin by first looking at the amazing digestive system.

Everything that is ingested and processed in the digestive tract becomes more than macronutrients (carbohydrates, fats and protein), it becomes a sea of chemicals, minerals, enzymes, beneficial bacteria and vitamins, many of which modern research is still exploring. These chemicals make up every structure, reaction and function within the human body. Because of this you cannot separate one organ system from another—if blood flows to it, then the food you eat and the chemicals contained in that food go there too.

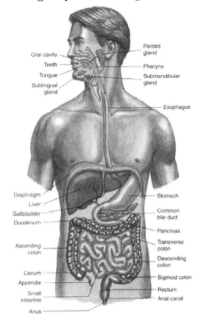

Every culture on the planet has its own distinct food history; as man evolved, they learned from observation which foods were safe, satisfying, strengthening and enlightening (ceremonial foods). Because of this, each population evolved the ability to digest and utilize foods unique to its environment.

We are dependent on the digestive system to process and absorb nutrients regardless of whether they come from nutraceuticals or natural whole foods.[28] The digestive system is made up of multiple organs: the mouth, pharynx, esophagus, stomach, small and large intestine, liver, gallbladder, pancreas, kidneys and bladder. [29, 30]

The word "digestion" means "to take apart"; it is the process whereby food is broken down mechanically and chemically in the gastrointestinal tract and converted into absorbable forms.

In 2013, research papers began appearing using the term "Leaky Gut Syndrome" as though it were a new discovery. Leaky Gut Syndrome is used to describe intestinal or bowel hyperpermeability. Tight junctions represent the major barrier within the pathway between intestinal epithelial cells that line the digestion tract. These

[28] Digestive Wellness, Elizabeth Lipski, PhD, CCN
[29] (Ross, 2000) Pg 330
[30] (Tabers, 2001) Pg 599

junctions become weak and no longer effectively control bowel permeability, and epithelial cells lose their protective function.

Minerals, water and monosaccharides can be absorbed as-is by the digestive tract and directly taken up into the bloodstream. Fats, starches and proteins, however, must be broken down into smaller molecules.[31]

Digestion and absorption is virtually impossible without enzymes. Enzymes are the essential building blocks of life. They are the key to the body's ability to properly digest and benefit from the foods we eat. Enzymes provide the energy we need to rebuild muscles, cells, nerves, tissues, bones and glands. They spark the chemical reactions responsible for breathing, digestion, growth and reproduction.[32] They are currently being studied for their role in anti-aging and cognition.[33]

Definition Of Enzymes

Enzymes are proteins that act as catalysts, speeding the rate of biochemical reactions. Enzymes are found in every cell of every living plant, microorganism and animal, including humans. They can only be formed from organic living matter. Enzymes are required for the healthy functioning of every organ system. They direct, accelerate, modify or retard all body functions. They do so in a unique, step-by-step, highly efficient, safe and remarkably economical manner.

Enzymes serve as the body's labor force and help perform every single function required for our daily activities. They also support our immune system. As biocatalysts, they either begin a reaction or cause a reaction to speed up. Without enzymes, life would not exist.

Enzymatic Process

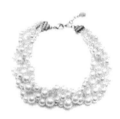

Enzymes work by virtue of their shape. Enzyme molecules can be compared in shape to short lengths of pearls (amino acids) strung and wound together. This long string folds in on itself as certain sequences of amino acids are more attracted to each other than to other sequences, thus giving the enzymes a specific shape. At one point on the surface of

---

[31] (Tabers, 2001) Pg 599-600
[32] (Howard F. Loomis, 1999)
[33] http://www.nutraingredients-usa.com/Consumer-Trends/Huge-opportunities-in-the-emerging-cognitive-health-market-Enzymotec-USA-CEO

the string of "pearls" there is something resembling a keyhole. This is called the active site on the enzyme. When matched with its particular coenzyme (vitamin, mineral or trace elements), this "lock" accepts the key contained in the molecule of the enzyme's substrate. The molecular structure is transformed into a different structure; both the enzymes and the newly transformed molecule are free to part.[34]

Dr. Max Wolf, MD, researched enzymes and hormones at Columbia University from the 1930s through the 1960s. Dr. Wolf determined that enzyme production diminishes in humans after age 27. Humans have historically supplemented their enzyme levels by consuming fresh, raw foods. Modern preservation and preparation techniques often destroy the enzymes these foods contain. This is the basis of the currently popular raw food diet.[35]

Enzyme deficiency can cause the body's functions to become less efficient. And yet, in the past, the medical establishment paid only limited attention to this vital biological component. When enzymes were traditionally studied in medical school, the emphasis was placed primarily on their digestive functions in the pancreas and gastrointestinal tract.[36] Sports medicine has taken the lead on using proteolytic enzymes for injuries and for the reduction of inflammation and scar tissue.

Clinicians used to be taught that oral enzymes were indicated only for digestive problems and not for any other medical conditions, as they were not readily absorbed. Unfortunately, in the United States and in other countries this was generally accepted as medical dogma and the potential importance of enzymes for other conditions was overlooked for decades.

In addition to being used for digestive disorders, enzymes are now widely utilized to treat various types of blood clots (particularly those causing heart attacks and occlusions of the leg veins), cancer, allergies, chronic inflammatory illnesses and several congenital deficiency diseases.[37]

Systemic Enzymes vs. Digestive Enzymes

Digestive enzymes help digest food in the small intestine. Systemic or proteolytic enzymes are programmed to survive stomach acid and to activate at only the right pH level. These enzymes need to be taken on an empty stomach to direct their

---

[34] (D.A. Lopez, 1994)
[35] The Raw Truth, Jordan Rubin, 2010
[36] (Anthony J. Cichoke, 1994)
[37] (D.A. Lopez, 1994)

action toward reducing inflammation, not aiding digestion. In this way they can pass through the stomach into the small intestines, where they are activated and can be absorbed into the bloodstream. Serrapeptase, commonly used for chronic pain, is also known as Serratia peptidase. This proteolytic enzyme is used in Europe and Asia instead of NSAIDs and as an alternative to aspirin and ibuprofen.[38]

Clinicians and patients need to remember that enzymes speed activity. This is especially important for those who are taking pharmaceutical medications like Coumadin and prescription painkillers. Enzymatic activity can work so strongly on the medicine's efficacy that it can be as if you had doubled the dosage. Proteolytic enzymes may help increase the impact of pain medication without having to take additional pills. DO NOT take medications and enzymes simultaneously and DO NOT attempt this without the supervision of your pain specialist.

Benefits of Systemic Proteolytic Enzymes

- Supplementation speeds recovery from exercise and injury
- Prevents the buildup of excessive fibrin and scar tissue
- Digests dead tissue, blood clots, cysts and arterial plaque
- Reduces inflammation, speeds healing from bruises and other tissue injuries including fractures, and reduces overall recovery time
- Unblocks arteries in coronary patients

Probiotics

The immune system comprises all structures and processes that are involved in defending against outside entities that attempt to infiltrate or degrade any part of the body. Specifically, it involves anatomic barriers such as the skin and mucous membranes which physically block the entry of antigens into the body, and physiological barriers (body temperature and acidity) that inhibit the growth of or kill detrimental microorganisms, as well as the various organs and cells of the immune system itself. The overall coordination of the immune system takes place in the hypothalamus and pineal glands.

---

[38] (William Wong, 2003)

When the digestive tract becomes compromised by poor eating habits, stress, chemicals, environmental toxins and/or heavy metals, the health of the entire body jeopardized. Our immune system protects us, not only from viruses, bacteria and yeasts, but also from naturally occurring mutant cells that can evolve into cancer.

Beneficial microorganisms, or probiotics, are small organisms that are beneficial to human health and are too small to be visible to the naked eye. An imbalance in the ratio of beneficial microorganisms and detrimental microorganisms in the body is known as dysbiosis. Probiotics comprise approximately 90% of the digestive tract bacteria in healthy persons.[39, 40]

Probiotics in the colon can lower total serum cholesterol levels, which helps heal ulcerative colitis and urinary tract infections (UTIs) by producing hydrogen peroxide (which is utilized by the body to "extinguish" neutralized antigen/antibody complexes). In the colon, probiotics ferment insoluble fiber, starch and undigested carbohydrates. The short-chain saturated fatty acids produced by this fermentation are the principal source of energy for the epithelial cells of the colon.[41, 42, 43] In addition, probiotics manufacture vitamins that not only help with energy and nerve function[44] but are necessary for brain health[45]: biotin, choline, folic acid, inositol, PABA (para aminobenzoic acid), vitamin B2, vitamin B5, vitamin B6 and vitamin K.

According to a new study, probiotics are effective in preventing hepatic encephalopathy in patients with cirrhosis of the liver. The investigators conducted trials with cirrhosis patients who showed risk factors for hepatic encephalopathy, but had yet to experience an obvious episode. When comparing treatment with probiotics versus placebo, the researchers found that the incidence of hepatic encephalopathy was lower in patients treated with probiotics.[46]

Fructooligosaccharides (FOS) are considered a soluble fiber and a prebiotic that support the growth of beneficial microorganisms in the intestinal tract while

[39] (In-Tele-Health)

[40] (Tabers, 2001)

[41] Norwich BioScience Institutes. "How bacteria with a sweet tooth may keep us healthy." ScienceDaily. ScienceDaily, 25 October 2013. <www.sciencedaily.com/releases/2013/10/131025185704.htm>.

[42] Norwich BioScience Institutes. "Sticky solution for identifying effective probiotics." ScienceDaily. ScienceDaily, 25 November 2009. <www.sciencedaily.com/releases/2009/11/091124113611.htm>

[43] Wiley. "Probiotics prevent diarrhea related to antibiotic use, review shows." ScienceDaily. ScienceDaily, 30 May 2013. <www.sciencedaily.com/releases/2013/05/130530192404.htm>.

[44] Wiley-Blackwell. "A gut-full of probiotics for your neurological well-being." ScienceDaily. ScienceDaily, 5 July 2011. <www.sciencedaily.com/releases/2011/07/110705210737.htm>.

[45] University of Michigan Health System. "Probiotics reduce stress-induced intestinal flare-ups, study finds." ScienceDaily. ScienceDaily, 14 March 2013. <www.sciencedaily.com/releases/2013/03/130314110256.htm>.

[46] American Gastroenterological Association. "Probiotics prevent deadly complications of liver disease, study finds." ScienceDaily. ScienceDaily, 6 June 2014. <www.sciencedaily.com/releases/2014/06/140606102047.htm>.

inhibiting the growth of harmful bacteria. FOS provide nourishment to most types of beneficial bacteria (because beneficial bacteria are living organisms they require nutrition like any living organism). Note that FOS is NOT a source of nourishment for toxic bacteria.

Pharmaceutical antibiotics destroy the body's beneficial bacteria in addition to any detrimental bacteria. Long-term usage (e.g., more than one month) of grapefruit seed extract, large amounts of raw garlic, goldenseal, silver protein and pasteurized foods have been found to destroy the body's endogenous probiotics in the digestive tract.

Ideally, retailers of beneficial bacteria products should keep their products refrigerated up to the point of sale (beneficial bacteria die at a much faster rate when they are not refrigerated). A recent survey conducted by the National Nutritional Foods Association (USA) found that 50% of beneficial bacteria supplements in retail stores contained significantly fewer viable beneficial bacteria than claimed on the label. Freeze-dried (lyophilized) beneficial bacteria supplements, usually in the form of powder, have a longer shelf-life than non-freeze-dried products.

Caution should be exercised when recommending probiotic products grown in a yeast matrix. It has been my clinical experience that these products can increase yeast overgrowth (thrush, athlete's foot, jock itch and vaginal irritation) in clients with candida albicans overgrowth.

What's Your pH?

I'm frequently asked what I think of acid/alkaline balancing plans. This particular protocol has a remarkable and interesting history that is not widely known.

The Alkaline diet™ is based on the theory that certain foods, when consumed, leave an alkaline residue, or ash. Minerals like calcium, iron, magnesium, zinc and copper are said to be the principle components of the ash. A food is thus classified as alkaline, acid or neutral according to the pH of the solution created with its ash in water.

A Little History

In 1863, Dr. James Caleb Jackson operated the Dansville Sanitarium in Dansville, New York. Dr. Jackson was a staunch vegetarian. One of Dr. Jackson's patrons was Ellen G. White. Ms. White went on to found the Seventh Day Adventist religion which advocates a vegetarian lifestyle. One of the members of Sister White's new church was John Kellogg.

Dr. John Harvey Kellogg's vocation was in the health spa and hospital business. He was the superintendent of Battle Creek Sanitarium in Battle Creek, Michigan. While history has relegated John Kellogg's medical status to that of "bowel-obsessed" quack (as noted in the novel and film, *Road to Wellville*), in his day he was considered a very skilled surgeon. He was a very devout man and is also known for his development of the Religion of Biologic Living.[47]

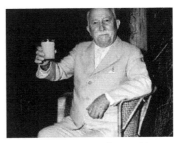

Dr. John Harvey Kellogg at his
Sanitarium in Battle Creek;
www.discovery.com

Charles William Post entered the Battle Creek Sanitarium in February of 1893 to recover from a second nervous breakdown. While recuperating, he became impressed with the new-fangled "health" foods being served. The stay at the sanitarium didn't do much for Post's health, but it did revive a passing interest in food development. The following year, he founded his own sanitarium, La Vita Inn.

All of this took place during the Victorian era, which is known for producing idiosyncratic views about health as well as morality.

Dr. Kellogg, for example, believed that sexual relations were not only sinful but detrimental to one's health. He reported that he and his wife had been married for over forty years and had never once "polluted" themselves with fornication. He later went on to say that he had 100% success with his patients. Any who were not cured, he claimed, must have foiled their own recovery because of "self-pollution" (sex or masturbation) and/or because they ate "animal flesh"—actions which were, to his mind, both sinful and the cause of disease.

A somewhat similar diet, the Hay diet, was developed by the American physician William Howard Hay in the 1920s. Another theory, called "nutripathy", was developed by American Gary A. Martin in the 1970s. Others who have advocated alkaline-acid balancing diets include D.C. Jarvis, Robert Young, Herman Aihara, Fred Shadian and Victor A. Marcial-Vega.

---

[47] http://www.amazon.com/Harvey-Kellogg-Religion-Biologic-Living/dp/0253014476/ref=pd_sim_sbs_b_1?ie=UTF8&refRID=00AMH5K1T99PXZ7S4Y1P

Today

The pH Miracle by Robert O. Young, PhD, and Shelley Redford Young is currently one of the most well-known books on the subject and is frequently brought in to my office by curious clients. It suggests a strict vegetarian eating plan. In my view, its protocol does not hold up in light of cutting edge research in nutrigenomics, cancer nutrition sciences and phytochemical studies.

Another popular book on the subject is *The Acid-Alkaline Diet* by Dr. Christopher Vasey, a Swiss naturopath. It recommends a vegetarian, predominately raw food lifestyle and restricts the consumption of grain, sugar, fruit, dairy, eggs, mushrooms, alcohol, caffeine, condiments, fermented foods, fat, nuts and even many vegetables. Both Dr. Young and Dr. Vasey claim that one can obtain all the protein necessary for muscle, tissue, bone and brain health from vegetable sources like soy. [48, 49]

For some, this protocol may be somewhat beneficial if they are highly sensitive to sugars, gluten, yeasts and molds. One may feel better when these items are restricted due to the elimination of inflammatory agents. Also, weight loss can occur because of what is called a catabolic state, which results in the destruction of cells, tissues and hormones; basically, one is feeding off of their own body. Foods such as broccoli, berries, organic meats and fish oils have been proven to be effective in preventing cancer, heart disease, depression and diabetes. Please don't end up eliminating healthy foods because you think it will balance your pH.

From 1920-1945, Dr. Weston A. Price conducted extensive anthropologic studies on indigenous populations, searching not only for the cause of degenerative illnesses but also for the perfect vegetarian diet. He never found an indigenous population who was vegetarian. Dr. Price's research took him to every continent. He consistently found that it was not the meat, fat, dairy or fruit that individuals ate that created health issues; rather, it was processed foods and refined sugars, grains, fats and salt that rapidly damaged the human body (*Nutrition and Physical Degeneration*, Weston A. Price).

The research conducted by Dr. Price and his team in the 1920s and 1930s would be difficult, if not impossible, for us to recreate today. First, the populations he studied lived in remote areas that were untouched by modern lifestyles; today it is unlikely that such a vast collection of indigenous populations exist. Additionally, the research methodology would be difficult to replicate and it may not satisfy modern ethical

---

[48] (Robert O. Young, 2005)
[49] (Rubin, 2010)

standards—just as Dr. Keys' work with conscientious objectors and low-calorie diets in the 1940s would not likely to be able to be reproduced today. [50]

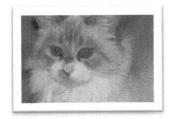

If we did nothing more than take high-quality digestive and proteolytic enzymes, we would reduce our likelihood of developing many age-related illnesses. Francis M. Pottenger, Jr., MD (1901–1967), conducted from 1932-42 what is known as the Pottenger Cat Study. In 1940, Pottenger purchased cottages from the Monrovia sanatorium and founded the Francis M. Pottenger, Jr. Hospital. Until it closed in 1960, the 42-bed hospital specialized in treating non-tubercular diseases of the lung, especially asthma.

Dr. Pottenger's longitudinal study of nutrients and what is now recognized as the enzymes present in raw foods was decades ahead of its time.

According to the Price-Pottenger Nutrition Foundation, "one particular question Pottenger addressed in his study had to do with the nutritive value of heat-labile elements — nutrients destroyed by heat and available only in raw foods. He applied the principles of nutrition and endocrinology early in his practice. Dr. Pottenger was a pioneer in using crude extracts of adrenal cortex as supplements to treat allergic states and exhaustion. In his treatment of respiratory diseases such as TB, asthma, allergies and emphysema, he always highlighted proper diet based on the principles discovered by Weston Price. At his hospital, he served liberal amounts of liver, butter, cream and eggs to convalescing patients." [51]

The "Pottenger's cats study" has been forgotten or overlooked by many in the current medical establishment. The study clearly supports eating real, natural foods loaded with enzymes to prevent degeneration and illness.

Minerals and enzymes are the two most important biochemical elements utilized by our body. They are vital to healthy cell replication and stabilize the delicate pH balance of the blood, saliva, urine and tissues. Without enzymes, we won't live very long. The complex phytochemicals found in fruits and vegetables interact with cell mitochondria to maintain healthy cell replication and energy. The only way to achieve good health is surprisingly straightforward: clean up your diet and go back to eating real foods that don't come out of boxes, cans, bottles and plastic bags.

---

[50] http://www.bcmj.org/article/ancel-keys-and-lipid-hypothesis-early-breakthroughs-current-management-dyslipidemia
[51] http://en.wikipedia.org/wiki/Francis_M._Pottenger,_Jr.

I routinely remind my clients that if their great-great-grandmother wouldn't recognize the ingredients on the label, don't eat or buy it. We shouldn't need a biochemistry degree to shop for food.

The Liver

Most of us spend very little time thinking about our liver. Much attention is focused on the heart and the brain, and for good reason, but the liver is equally as important.

Where is the liver in relation to everything else? If you're an anatomy student, you can probably lay your hand right on it. The liver is located under the bottom ribs on the right side of the abdomen and only inches from the heart, kidneys and gut. The liver is the largest internal organ and the second largest next to the skin. It comprises 2.5% of total body weight and is the only organ able to regenerate after injury or illness. The liver participates in functions associated with the cardiovascular, digestive and excretory systems and also plays a role in metabolism.

The liver stores and filters the blood to remove infectious organisms. It processes approximately three pints of blood every minute. Most blood arrives at the liver directly from the intestines via the portal vein carrying dietary nutrients and toxins. The remaining blood arrives at the liver via the hepatic artery. The liver is the primary organ for detoxification of toxic chemicals that enter the body through skin, respiration and ingestion; it is responsible for the metabolism of 90% of ingested alcohol and 25% of basal metabolism and for the conversion of stored glycogen into glucose for release into the bloodstream.

Geneticists have discovered that approximately 40% of the population are poor methylaters. These individuals have difficulty collecting and utilizing nutrients like B vitamins and sulfur compounds that aid in conversion to co-factors. It is entirely possible that this is also the cause of reduced carbohydrate metabolism, which would also affect the liver's ability to control glycogen, leptin, and cholesterol production and utilization. Could this be part of the reason for the pandemic increases in diabetes and non-alcoholic fatty liver disease? Time will tell us more.

If your liver is bogged down with high fructose corn sweetener, medications and chemicals you are increasing your risk factors for type 2 diabetes, fatty liver disease, hormone disruption and obesity.

For those with thyroid disease, approximately 80% of triiodothyronine (T3) is produced in the liver from the conversion of thyroxine (T4) to T3 and T3 accounts for 20% of thyroid hormone production. Triiodothyronine (T3) is approximately ten times more potent than thyroxine (T4). A healthy liver is central to hormone production and utilization of all hormones: insulin, testosterone, progesterone, estrogens (there are more than one), melatonin, DHEA and others.

The liver stores several vitamins and minerals for the body to use including cobalt, 15% of the body's copper, manganese, ferritin (the endogenous form of iron), coenzyme Q10, biotin and folic acid. Vitamins A, C, D, E, K, B1, B2, B5, B6 and B12 all concentrate in the liver. But that's not all; endogenous phospholipids (healthy fats), and proteins are manufactured in the liver as well as cholesterol, which protects the brain, heart and hormones.

> ## Ailments Caused by Liver Malfunction
> Liver malfunction may cause adult acne, rosacea, halitosis (bad breath) and psoriasis.

Intestinal permeability may be an underlying cause of liver malfunction. This can occur due to the additional workload placed on the liver of detoxifying antigens that enter the body as a result of poor gut health. This is an especially important consideration for children and adults with gluten sensitivity and autism spectrum. Systemic lupus erythematosus (SLE), a form of the serious autoimmune disease lupus erythematosus (LE), and hepatitis A, B and C infections cause degeneration and death of the liver. Additional impaired liver function may occur as a result of adrenal insufficiency and gluten sensitivity.

People with liver ailments should avoid carnitine, "smart drugs" (Adrafinil, Propranolol only with caution), Xanthinol Nicotinate, the herbs coltsfoot , licorice, and valerian, and high iron-containing foods such as watermelon, strawberries, sesame seeds, pumpkin seeds, liver, molasses and prunes.

People with liver ailments should consume herbs such as artichoke leaf, green tea, jiaogulan, Korean ginseng, lycium and milk thistle as well as black cherry (juice), grape (juice), lemon (juice, drink upon awakening in the morning), pear (juice) and reishi mushrooms. Many of these herbs and foods are found in high-quality liver detox products and plans.

I encourage you to do a liver detox twice a year and to follow in the footsteps of your ancestors by eating grass-fed, organically raised liver one to four times a month (if you do not have hepatitis C or elevated ferritin levels). Liver is nature's multi-vitamin, and eating liver helps your liver to be healthier. Our ancestors knew this. It's time to return to those old-fashioned food values that kept all of us healthier.

Gallbladder, Workmate Of The Liver

Did you know that you can have gallbladder stones *after* having your gallbladder removed? You can still develop stones in the ducts that lead to the gallbladder from the liver.

While getting gallstones after a cholecystectomy (removal of the gallbladder) is rare, it can occur and will require medical treatment. To understand how gallstones can return after gallbladder surgery, it is essential to comprehend the function of the gallbladder and how gallstones are formed.

Your gallbladder is a small pear-shaped organ in the abdomen and holds a digestive fluid called bile, which is made up of 70% cholesterol. People suffering from gallbladder disease or who have recently had gallstone surgery may benefit from following a low-fat and low-cholesterol diet;[52, 53] family history should also be considered.

Located just under the liver, the gallbladder is connected by the common bile duct to the liver. The liver produces bile that drains into the gallbladder, which serves as a reservoir. When we consume food, the gallbladder contracts and releases the bile through the common bile duct, which travels into the small intestine. Bile is a fluid-like substance that helps digest the fats in the foods we consume.

Cholesterol in the bile forms stone-like deposits that can range in size from a tiny grain of sand to the size of a golf ball. These deposits are known as gallstones. While almost everyone has gallstones, a portion of the population will develop complications from having these deposits. These complications occur when the gallstones block or become lodged in the duct, blocking the flow of bile. These stones can also form in the bile ducts. This condition, known as choledocholithiasis, can cause the stones to travel and block the pancreatic duct if left untreated.

---

[52] http://www.livestrong.com/article/346199-diet-after-gallstone-surgery/
[53] http://www.helium.com/items/1169768-gallstones-after-having-the-gallbladder-removed

Symptoms can include minor to severe pain in the upper abdomen, upper back pain, nausea and/or vomiting. Often, individuals believe they are experiencing indigestion and do not seek medical attention until the pain becomes unbearable.[54]

Bile aids in the digestion of fats. After the gallbladder has been removed, the body may not produce enough bile to properly digest fats, resulting in upset stomach and diarrhea. To help prevent this, avoid hydrogenated oils, margarine, saturated fats and fried foods. You should not eliminate all fats from your diet. Healthy fats such as olive oil and omega-3 fatty acids should be included in small amounts as the body benefits from these healthy fats.

Fiber, with proper fluid intake, moves through the digestive tract with little effort, helping to keep the tract free of blockages. High-fiber choices include whole-wheat pasta, oatmeal, split peas, lentils and black beans. According to the Mayo Clinic, you should try to consume 25 to 38 grams of fiber per day.

After the gallbladder has been removed, a diet that includes plenty of fresh, organic fruits and vegetables is beneficial to help you heal. In addition to providing fiber, fresh fruits and vegetables are naturally low in fat and contain valuable vitamins and minerals. Recommended fruits and vegetables include beets, cucumbers, onions, garlic, grapes, lemons, tomatoes, apples and berries. [55, 56, 57]

The Mayo Clinic recommends taking a vitamin supplement due to deficiencies in vitamin C, vitamin E or calcium may cause you to experience digestive discomfort. You can add turmeric and ginger to meals to aid in bile production and fat digestion. When dining at restaurants, keep dressing off of salads, select grilled chicken or fish, and order rice or potatoes without butter and sour cream.

---

[54] http://voices.yahoo.com/preventing-gallstones-after-gallbladder-removal-2102510.html
[55] http://www.livestrong.com/article/346199-diet-after-gallstone-surgery/
[56] http://www.webmd.com/digestive-disorders /open-gallbladder-surgery-for-gallstones
[57] http://www.gastromdg astromd.com/education/bileductstones.html

Vitamins were discovered not because of idle curiosity, but because of the scourge of disease. In 1905, William Fletcher was the first scientist to determine that if special factors (later dubbed "vitamins") were removed from food, illness and disease soon followed. Dr. Fletcher was searching for the cause of beriberi when he discovered that eating unpolished rice prevented beriberi because it contained vitamin B1 (thiamin).

In 1912, the Polish scientist Casimir Funk named the nutritional parts of food "vitamine" after *vita* meaning life and *amine* from compounds found in the thiamine he isolated from rice husks. Together, Hopkins and Funk formulated the vitamin hypothesis of deficiency disease: a lack of vitamins could make you sick. [58, 59]

When we look at a seed such as wheat or rice we find several layers. It is within these layers that Casimir Funk found the nutrients he later named vitamins. The layers are comprised of the **bran** (the outer "wrapper")which contains lots of fiber

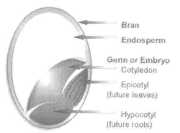

and minerals such as iron and vitamin B_1; the **germ** or embryo which contains many of the B vitamins and the fat-soluble vitamins like vitamin A, D and E, a number of minerals, and high quality protein; and the **endosperm**, which is mostly short-chain starch, a small quantity of low-quality protein, and almost no vitamins or minerals.

When wheat is milled into white flour, the bran and germ are removed, leaving only the endosperm. These isolated short-chain starches are readily converted to sugar, creating dangerous blood sugar surges for diabetics and hypoglycemics. When the leftover endosperm is further chemically treated (bleached) to make it appear even whiter, more nutrients are destroyed. This pre-digested starch is believed by some researchers to play a role in fatty liver disease as it can easily pass through the gut directly into the liver with little or no digestive action beyond freeing up the saccharides it contains.

Hildegard of Bingen, a 12th century abbess, poet, author, mystic, musician and renowned healer, whose work *Physica* has been translated into English by Priscilla Throop, reminds us that processed wheat has been known for centuries to be

---

[58] (Bellis, 2011)
[59] (Carter, 1996)

harmful to human health. She wrote, "If anyone sifts out the bran from the flour, and then makes bread from that flour, the bread is weaker and more feeble than if it had been made from the proper flour. Without its bran, the flour loses its strength somewhat, and produces more mucous in a person than that made from the whole wheat flour.

Whosoever cooks grain, or wheat without the entire grain, or wheat not ground in the mill, it is as if he eats another food, for this wheat furnishes neither correct blood nor healthy flesh, but more mucous. It is scarcely digested."

In 1943, the United States government admitted that modern processing might cause nutritional deficiencies. So, by law, manufacturers of white flour must manually add back three specific B vitamins (thiamine or B_1, riboflavin or B_2, and niacin or B_3) and iron. Thus, the bleached white flour is "enriched". Unprocessed whole wheat contains around 16 minerals and 11 vitamins that are mostly removed during processing, yet only these three synthetically produced vitamins and iron are all that must be added back in.

Carbohydrates

Carbohydrates are organic compounds of carbon, hydrogen and oxygen in which (with few exceptions), the ratio of hydrogen to oxygen is 2:1. The body uses carbohydrates as a source of energy and heat (after conversion to glucose via glycogen which subsequently reverts back to glucose). Dietary carbohydrates are initially converted to and stored as glycogen until their subsequent conversion to either glucose or adipose tissue (fat). Carbohydrates account for 1% of human body weight. The optimal human diet would consist of 60% carbohydrates, of which 45% would be polysaccharides and 15% would be simple sugars.[60]

The optimal total daily intake of carbohydrates is 75-150 grams per day (the present average consumption in Western nations is 250-400 grams per day). The FDA recommends a maximum daily intake of 300-375 grams of dietary carbohydrates. Could an over-consumption of carbohydrates account for our ever-increasing waistlines and epidemic of mood disorders? Remember, more carbohydrates equals more calories, many of which come from refined #2 field corn products like high fructose corn sweetener.

---

[60] (In-Tele-Health)

Carbohydrates come in all colors, sizes and shapes. The rich, buttery orange of a winter squash is due to the healthy carotenoids that are activated by cooking. The sweet tang of bing cherries, the refreshing zest of savory herbs; these flavorful foods do not elevate blood sugars and the flavonoids present reduce inflammation in the joints and muscle tissues like the heart.

In general, the fresher your fruits and vegetables are, the higher their nutrition quality. If you are overweight or diabetic, your health will generally improve if you select vegetables low on the glycemic scale like cherries, berries, mixed greens, beans, fennel, onion, garlic and asparagus. The carbohydrates that have the highest impact on blood sugars are considered starches: corn, potatoes, squash, rice and wheat. Also, fruits like melon, pineapple, banana and mango can lead to a spike in blood sugar, increasing insulin levels that lead to inflammation.

Alcohol will rapidly convert to sugar and elevate blood glucose levels. This and the foods mentioned above should be consumed only occasionally and in limited quantities by individuals who are trying to lose weight or who have heart disease or diabetes. This is due to the hormone insulin. The more insulin levels rise to meet the increase in blood sugar, the more inflammation affects your body, increasing your risk of heart disease, type 2 diabetes and inflammatory illnesses.[61, 62, 63]

The more processed a carbohydrate is, the faster it will have adverse effects on the body. Three saltine crackers will elevate a diabetic's blood sugars faster than table sugar. This is because the flour in the crackers has been refined to almost pure glucose, which can be absorbed quickly through the mucous membranes of the mouth and throat. Breads made of white or whole wheat flours will also convert rapidly, bouncing blood sugar levels up and down like a yo-yo. Often, sugars and starches are added that the body does not know what to do with, like high fructose corn sweetener (HFCS).

The liver manufactures the hormone leptin which signals to the brain when you are eating and when you are getting full. HFCS (high fructose corn sweetener) blocks this hormone and the brain fails to get the signal you have eaten or consumed calories. Twenty years after leptin was found to regulate metabolism and weight through brain cells called neurons, researchers have found the hormone also acts on other types of cells to control appetite.

---

[61] (Diana Schwarzbein, 1999)

[62] (Daoust, 2001)

[63] (Diana Schwazbein, 2004)

Leptin is also known for its hunger-blocking effect on the hypothalamus, a region in the brain. Food intake is influenced by signals that travel from the body to the brain. Leptin is one of the molecules that signal the brain to modulate food intake.[64]

Research shows that a woman at age 40 and above who consumes one 12 oz. soft drink daily (made with HFCS) increases her diabetes risk factors by 50 percent. HFCS is one of the most insidious chemicals placed in our food since 1980. Obesity and diabetes rates have sky-rocketed over the same 29-year time period that the food industry has switched from using sugar to using HFCS.

In 2009, the corn product manufacturers of America started an ad campaign to protect their production of HFCS. These ads informed consumers that HFCS was no different from sugar and that as long as it was consumed in moderation it was no more harmful than regular sugar (and they claimed that dieticians concurred). By the end of 2010, the corn industry had made the decision to discontinue the use of the name high fructose corn sweetener and changed it to corn sugar. Nothing has changed but the name; your liver still has the potential of being damaged by this chemically derived sweetener.

Antioxidants

They come in a rainbow of colors: purple, red, orange, yellow and green. They are the antioxidant-rich foods that keep us healthy. Studies over the last three decades have shown that this group of nutrients can protect against cancers, cataracts, macular degeneration, allergies, heart disease, inflammatory diseases and more than 80 age-related illnesses. They can also slow the aging process.

Antioxidants make up a growing group of minerals, herbs and vitamins, such as vitamins C, A and E; beta-carotene; bioflavonoids; selenium, germanium, lycopene and proanthocyanidins. They are found in all fruits and vegetables, and it is easy to use food concentrates or nutraceuticals to ensure adequate intake of disease-fighting antioxidants.

---

[64] Yale University. "Leptin also influences brain cells that control appetite, researchers find." ScienceDaily. ScienceDaily, 1 June 2014. <www.sciencedaily.com/releases/2014/06/140601150930.htm>.

A Little History

The free radical theory of aging was first described in 1954 by Dr. Denham Harman. He stated that "a single common process, modifiable by genetic and environmental factors, was responsible for aging and death in all living things." He continues, "Aging is caused by free radical reactions, which may be caused by the environment, from disease and intrinsic reactions within the aging process."

It has taken 55 years for Dr. Harman's work to be taken seriously by the medical community. The conventional wisdom stated that disease must come from outside man, not as a by-product of normal biological functions. Many still do not fully understand the importance of antioxidants in the prevention of disease.

Nutrigenomics studies are showing that the best way to obtain antioxidants is via whole foods. On a cellular level, whole foods interface with DNA in an extremely efficient manner. Isolated nutrients, in contrast, may have little or no effect on mitochondrial energy function.

Free Radicals

No matter how many antioxidants we consume, there will always be some free radical production. Free radical production is normal and occurs every time we breathe in air, eat food or place products on our skin. Some common triggers include:

- ✓ Stress: Emotional or physical; makes you breathe less and burn more energy. Stress feeds on anaerobic metabolism, not oxygen.
- ✓ Ozone in the air: Great way to produce superoxide.
- ✓ Auto exhaust: You breathe carbon monoxide and hydrochloric acid instead of oxygen.
- ✓ Cigarette and wood smoke: Same as auto exhaust.
- ✓ Inflammation: Your body's immune system creates free radicals to fight germs.
- ✓ Radiation: Alters molecules so they throw off free radicals.
- ✓ Sunlight: A form of radiation; *necessary for vitamin D production.*
- ✓ Contaminated water: Heavy metals, medications, petroleum, herbicides and pesticides are commonly found in municipal water supplies (what comes out of your tap). Be aware that store-bought bottled water may be nothing more than minimally filtered city water.

- ✓ Processed foods: Processed foods shift your body into anaerobic metabolism to try and get something useful out of the fake food you just consumed.
- ✓ Toxic metals and industrial chemicals: They are in the soil, water and air. Some professionals such as welders, fabricators, auto/aircraft detailers, herbicide applicators, gas station attendants, mechanics, janitors and landscapers have higher than average exposure rates.
- ✓ Drugs: They alter the body's ability to metabolize oxygen.

Antioxidant-Rich Foods

Here are just a few examples of antioxidant-rich foods: blueberries, cherries, raspberries, blackberries, greens, tomatoes, plums, peppers, grapes, winter squash, acai, pomegranate, beer, wine, spirulina, propolis, miso, tempeh, cranberries, kiwifruit, grapefruit, olives, oranges, lemons, limes, elderberries, mushrooms, herbs, cocoa, grape seeds, sesame seeds, green tea, garlic and onions. Alaskan salmon contain the antioxidant *astaxanthin* which comes from the krill the salmon feed on; this is what makes their flesh a bright red-pink in color.

There are hundreds of specialty nutraceuticals on the market designed to deliver targeted antioxidants that are not easily attainable from locally produced foods. Nutrient levels in foods vary from area to area based on soil condition, water and temperature. While in an ideal world, we should be able to gain all our nutrition from food, the reality is we may not be able to. Supplements are beneficial when they are from high-quality sources; they are recommended for anyone with chronic illness or cancer. However, if an individual is unwilling to make healthy food choices their health will continue to deteriorate. Supplements do not replace real food and it is impossible for the average person to eat enough real food to attain optimum antioxidants if they have predispositions towards a particular illness; therefore, supplementation may be called for. A support system which consists of nutrient-dense food, high-quality supplements and healthcare practitioners who are willing to develop a multifaceted health and wellness plan is the ideal solution.

Supplements: Vitamins, minerals, hormones and herbal products available over-the-counter at retail discount stores, mail-order companies and vitamin shops. These products can contain synthetic ingredients such as fillers, binders, artificial colors, flavorings and harmful chemicals like propylene glycol.

Additionally, potency may be reduced or lacking due to improper storage and manufacturer formulation.

Nutraceutical: Vitamins, minerals, hormones and herbal products that are certified organic and heavy metal-, gluten-, dairy-, soy- and contaminant-free. They are often referred to as "designer supplements".

Nutraceuticals are utilized by the body comparably to whole foods, where optimum bioavailability can occur on the mitochondria level. High-quality nutraceuticals provide support without overburdening the digestive system with potential carcinogens.

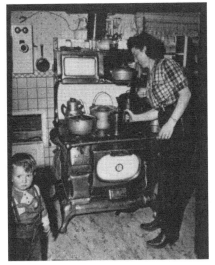

OHS image bb012655 – Lucille Meeks cooks a big meal on a woodstove for a branding party on her ranch near Bend, Oregon, in 1952.

Gas stoves, along with refrigerators and freezers, changed food preparation methods for individuals living on ranches in the eastern half of the Pacific Northwest following the development of the Bonneville Power Agency.

Regardless of your family history, genetic markers and personal living environment, food should always be your first medicine. Modern inventions have undoubtedly made food preparation and preservation more convenient, but it seems that as technology progresses, we seem more inclined to make our food the "*Star Trek* way" and may in some cases be sacrificing health for convenience.

A society which consumes lots of calories but little nutrients is headed for increased cancer risk, chronic illness, premature aging and more.

Chef Jamie Oliver recently began a campaign in Australia with the aim of encouraging people to learn how to prepare simple, fresh and healthy food. It was based on an initiative launched by the British government during the Second World War which aimed to educate the public on how to continue to eat healthily despite food rationing. Oliver's 10-week program was proven in a 2014 study to change peoples' attitudes towards food as well as their behavior. The research, published in the open access journal *BMC Public Health,* has found that these changes persist up to six months after completion of the program.[65]

Regardless of how hard Cargill® and Monsanto® try, genetically modified foods will not correctly insert into our RNA, which still resembles the RNA of Neolithic man. I frequently tell my clients, "Your cells carry the memories of your ancestors." If your great-great-great-grandmother wouldn't recognize the food on your plate or its core ingredients, then how do you expect your cells to?

---

[65] Jessica Herbert, Anna Flego, Lisa Gibbs, Elizabeth Waters, Boyd Swinburn, John Reynolds, Marj Moodie. Wider impacts of a 10-week community cooking skills program - Jamie's Ministry of Food, Australia. BMC Public Health, 2014; 14 (1): 1161 DOI: 10.1186/1471-2458-14-1161

For the prevention of breast and prostate health issues, the first thing I recommend is to avoid soy foods that are not fermented (and maybe even those that are) as soy contains phytoestrogens. If an individual is dealing with estrogen-driven breast health challenges, phytoestrogens are just as problematic as synthetic forms. A full 98% of the soy produced in the United States is genetically modified, as is the majority of corn. These food stuffs are banned in Japan as well as many other countries, because they read the complete study provided on the health risk assessment, unlike our Food and Drug Administration (the FDA decided to issue recommendations simply after reading the summary supplied by Monsanto®).

Flax, like soy, is another food that has gotten tremendous attention for its health properties. Did you know that linseed oil used in painting, is made by letting flax oil go rancid? When you read about flax and talk to those who are familiar with its use, you learn that flax oil used to be pressed fresh each day and delivered with the milk, butter and cream. Flax oil is so sensitive to heat, light and air that Dr. Udo Erasmus, one of the world's foremost experts on oils, designed and custom-ordered specialized equipment for pressing flax in order to achieve medicinal-quality oil. Flax, like soy, is a phytoestrogen and elevates estradiol levels in both men and women.

Minerals such as selenium are critical in cancer prevention. Three to four Brazil nuts contain the minimum daily recommendation of 200 mcg of selenium daily. It is not wise to go over 400 mcg of selenium daily without consulting a healthcare provider knowledgeable in nutrient protocols.

Mushrooms, dried or fresh, provide trace minerals and immune-building properties. Most breast, prostate, colon, stomach and liver health protocols call for the incorporation of mushrooms, providing you are not allergic or sensitive to them.

If you are worried about cancer of any kind, organic vegetables are a must. They are loaded with minerals, vitamins, phytonutrients, fiber and ingredients we don't have names for yet. Traditional herbalists will tell you that you can heal the body with herbs; many are now readily obtainable in the neighborhood supermarket, and farmers markets they are easily added to the evening meal.

One note on the cabbage family: steam or lightly cook these foods as they may cause digestive distress and slow thyroid function when consumed raw (although thyroid disruption is unlikely and may be based more on myth than fact). Cruciferous vegetable have the highest cancer-fighting properties when cooked or pickled. This could very well be why traditional dishes that incorporate the braccus family is usually pickled, fermented, steamed or cooked in some fashion. Grandmother really did know best.

Research now supports what holistic nutrition practitioners have always known: lean, organic protein is necessary for the body to heal and repair itself. Some individuals seem to do best with fish or poultry while others prefer lean red meats. Either way, 30 grams of protein is the current daily recommendation from noted oncologists Nicholas Gonzalez, MD and Thomas Cowan, MD. Not all proteins are created equal; if you are a vegetarian please seek the guidance of a qualified practitioner to ensure you are getting all the amino acids the body requires.

The United States, unlike other countries, does not have a single, longstanding food tradition. Our food history is a "mulligan stew" where one nationality's dietary traditions blend into another's. Here, we tend to view food as fuel or substance; we only "eat to live." We look to government agencies, health professionals, diet books, T.V. and commercial food vendors to tell us what to eat. The result is fast food chains, processed foods and no deep, abiding connection with food.

For many in the modern world, our senses of taste, smell and texture are now programmed to prefer processed and synthesized foods over the homegrown meals prepared by our mothers or grandparents. Food preparation, by and large, focuses on convenience and is modeled after examples set by authors like Peg Braken in the 1960s.

In the past, we ate in season. We enjoyed berries, peaches, greens and sweet peas in the spring. Summer brought us delicious tomatoes, melons, carrots, bitter greens, beans, sweet corn and onions. Fall provided us with more substantial fare like grains, squash and potatoes. The saying "everything has its season" is especially true of food.

Beans

There are over one thousand varieties of beans (also known as pulses or legumes). There are three main types of beans, snap, shell and dry. Some of the "Baby Boomer generation" may have earned summer money by picking pole or snap beans. No doubt the pickers participated in bean fights as the season wore on.

Beans were discovered to have existed 20,000 years ago. The lima and pinto were cultivated by Mexican and Peruvian civilizations more than 7,000 years ago. As these peoples migrated into North America, they brought beans with them. Spanish explorers, in turn, introduced beans to Europe in the 1500s. From there, the Spanish and Portuguese traders carried beans into Africa and Asia.

The United States is currently the sixth largest producer of dry beans after Brazil, India, China, Burma and Mexico. The top producing states are North Dakota and Michigan.

Great northern, pinto, garbanzo, peas and lentils—all have benefits for your health. Beans count nutritionally both as a vegetable and a protein source. They are rich in fiber, both soluble and insoluble, and so help promote regularity, lower cholesterol and blood pressure, and reduce cancer risk. Beans are an excellent source of potassium, folate, magnesium, manganese, molybdenum and the thiamine.

Dark beans, like black beans, are rich in antioxidants called *anthocyanins,* which are also found in grapes, blueberries, cherries and cranberries. Of the top twenty antioxidant foods, four of them are beans. Beans have been prescribed as a remedy for constipation for centuries. If you are one of the unfortunate ones who suffer from flatulence, you may have avoided this healthy food group. In our family we have found that soaking dry beans for twenty-four hours, then running them through a pressure canner into handy pint or quart jars, make them a fast food and a gas-free food.

To help your digestive system adjust to beans and reduce flatulence, start slow with small amounts such as ¼ to ½ cup serving. Gas is often the result of introducing fiber to a gut that is not used to working without it. Products like Beano™ and digestive enzymes are also useful in breaking down the fiber and protein, which reduces gas.

Refried beans are fast to make with pre-canned beans; use one stick organic salted butter in a cast iron skillet, add one quart canned pinto or black beans, warm and mash with a potato masher, and add Celtic sea salt to taste. Beans are great in stews and soups as well as in side dishes with rice and quinoa.

Research shows that those who eat beans regularly, more so than other foods, seem to live longer regardless of ethnicity. Europeans have been eating beans for several centuries and there are many diverse and tasty dishes reflecting various cultures. According to the 1999-2002 National Health Survey, bean eaters were less likely to be obese. There is also conclusive data linking bean consumption and heart health. One study of 16,000 middle-aged men followed for 25 years showed that higher bean consumption resulted in lower risk for heart disease by an astounding 82%.

The consumption of beans is also associated with the reduction of breast cancer in postmenopausal women. For those with type 2 diabetes, beans, due to their fiber content, are beneficial for lowering and controlling blood sugars. The daily recommendation for fiber intake for a diabetic is 50 grams. Beans make it easy to get fiber without having to drink "sludge".

Berries

My personal favorites are blackberries, but strawberries, raspberries, blueberries, currants, gooseberries, cranberries, huckleberries and marionberries have incredible health benefits as well.

All of these berries are low-glycemic, meaning they are great for diabetics; they also help prevent cancer and support heart and eye health. Strawberries help curb your appetite; they contain vitamin C and iron, so they can be a perfect food for those who struggle with anemia.

Strawberries have been described by The Fat Resistance Diet (FRD) as a fruit that can increase a hormone that stimulates metabolism, suppresses appetite, and controls blood sugar after starchy meals while inhibiting inflammation. This hormone that strawberries trigger, *adiponectin*, is the fat-burning hormone that works with the hormone leptin, the hormone responsible for weight regulation. Having high levels of adiponectin in the bloodstream has been shown to lower the risk of heart attack while lower levels of adiponectin are indicative of obesity.

Blackberries have been found to have the highest antioxidant capacity. They are rich in vitamin C, fiber, phytochemicals, tannins, flavonoids and catechins. Blackberries also help alleviate allergies as they stop the action of histamine. If you are out camping and you get burned, try gently rubbing blackberry leaves on the area to soothe the skin. Blackberries have been found in human cell studies to prevent lung, esophageal, liver and colon damage/cancer.

Blueberries have been held in high regard by Native Americans for centuries. They believed they possess magical powers and were sent by the "Great Spirit" to feed children during times of famine. They are native to North America, as are two other berries, cranberry and Concord grape. Blueberries are rich in antioxidants, phytochemicals and ellagic acid, a natural chemical that may inhibit tumor growth. Fresh or frozen blueberries contain the highest levels of anthocyanins, whereas dried contain almost none. Blueberries have been found to be supportive of brain health, cognition and memory. They are antibacterial and are beneficial to the urinary tract system. As with other berries, they have high cancer-fighting properties. Blueberries have also been found to be good for the heart and circulatory system.

Elderberries contain more vitamin C than any other fruit except rose hips and black currants. They also contain vitamin A as well as carotenoids, flavonoids, tannins, polyphenols and anthocyanins. These chemicals fight cancer, heart disease, diabetes, infection and inflammation. Since the time of Hippocrates, healers have been using elderberries as a diuretic and laxative, to treat stomach ailments, and to promote urinary tract health. Studies have shown elderberries can effectively prevent influenza and the common cold. They are also recommended to treat colitis; in one study, there was a 50% reduction in colon damage after one month.

Raspberries are similar to their cousins blackberries and strawberries. There are over 200 known species of raspberries. Xylitol, the sugar substitute, is made from raspberries. Blackberries and raspberries are bramble fruits which are fruits formed by the aggregation of several smaller fruits, called drupelets. Raspberries are a good source of vitamin C, fiber, selenium and phosphorus, and are rich in a variety of antioxidants and phytochemicals associated with cancer and diabetes prevention. They have been found to effectively prevent fatty liver disease and to reduce obesity. Freezing destroys much of the vitamin C in raspberries, so enjoy them fresh when possible.

A note on xylitol: Although this sweetener is extracted from natural sources, this does not necessarily mean the processed substance is healthy or safe. Some individuals have adverse reactions to xylitol due to it having an alcohol base.

Cranberries, along with blueberries and Concord grapes, are one of North America's three native fruits that are commercially grown. Cranberries were first used by Native Americans. Cranberries today are commercially grown throughout the northern part of the United States and are available in both fresh and processed forms.

Cranberries are commonly used to treat urinary tract infections. Their ability to protect the delicate lining of the bladder and the urethra from bacteria and damage from acidic properties of urine has been known for centuries. Stress, aging, hormonal imbalance and low water consumption all contribute to kidney and bladder issues.

Phytonutrients present in cranberries include phenolic acids, proanthocyanidins, anthocyanins, flavonoids and triterpenoids. They are also high in fiber, vitamin C and manganese, all of which are central to the maintenance of tissue elastin, cell permeability and tissue flexibility as well as being anti-inflammatory. In the vascular system, cranberries inhibit the formation of plaque on the vessel walls.

The essential nutrients in cranberries help prevent premature aging and degenerative conditions like dementia. Studies have confirmed that cranberries help prevent cancer, specifically breast, colon, prostate and lung cancer.

Incorporating nutrient-rich cranberries into your diet in the form of easy-to-make sauces, dried fruit and juice can promote overall health and longevity. Be aware that canned cranberry products and some commercial juices may contain added sugar and may be missing vital nutrients.

Organic Versus Conventional Cranberries

Supporters of the use of pesticides to grow cranberries claim that the pesticides are necessary since the bogs are rife with natural pests and the wetlands encourage fungi. The What's On My Food website reveals that there are 13 pesticides commonly found on conventional cranberries. Of these, three are known or probable carcinogens, six are suspected hormone disruptors, five are neurotoxins and one is a developmental or reproductive toxin; six are honeybee toxins.

Things To Consider

There is one contraindication for cranberries: If you suffer from kidney stones, especially calcium-oxalate stones, cranberries may exacerbate your condition.

Cranberry juice has enormous health benefits, but whole berries pack a much greater nutritional punch.

Rule 1: If it takes a chemistry set to make or a chemistry book to figure out, don't buy it.

Health Benefits Of Peaches & Plums

Peaches are originally from China. They belong to the genus Prunus and to the family of Rosaceae; their scientific name is Prunus persica. Technically, the peach is a "drupe", having similar features to other members of the family Prunus including plums, nectarine, almonds and damson.

Peaches are low in calories (100 grams provide 39 calories) and contain no saturated fats. They are packed with minerals and vitamins. The total measured antioxidant strength (ORAC value) of 100 grams of peach fruit is 1814 TE.

Fresh peaches are a moderate source of vitamin A and ß-carotene. ß-carotene is a pro-vitamin which converts into vitamin A in the body. Consumption of fruits rich in vitamin A is known to offer protection from lung and oral cavity cancers. Additionally, peaches contain potassium, fluoride and iron. Potassium is an important component of cell and body fluids that help regulate heart rate and blood pressure. Fluoride is a component of bones and teeth and helps to prevent dental caries. Fluoride found in foods (unlike what is found in oral health products) does not have harmful side effects. Iron is required for red blood cell formation.

Peaches contain health-promoting flavonoid polyphenolic antioxidants such as lutein, zea-xanthin and ß-cryptoxanthin. These compounds help protect against the oxygen-derived free radicals and reactive oxygen species (ROS) that play a role in aging and various disease processes.

Organic Versus Commercial

The fruits and vegetables listed by the Environmental Working Group (EWG) as "The Dirty Dozen" tested positive, when conventionally grown, for at least 47 different chemicals; some tested positive for as many as 67. For produce on the "dirty" list, you should definitely go organic—unless you relish the idea of consuming a chemical cocktail.

"The Dirty Dozen" list includes:[66]

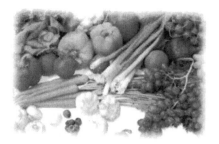

---

[66] http://www.ewg.org/foodnews/

celery

peaches

strawberries

apples

domestic blueberries

nectarines

sweet bell peppers

spinach, kale and collard greens

cherries

potatoes

imported grapes

lettuce

The produce on "The Clean 15" list contained none or negligible traces of pesticides and may be safe to consume in non-organic form. This list includes:

onions

avocados

pineapples

sweet peas

cabbage

cantaloupe

grapefruit

sweet onion

kiwi fruit

sweet corn

mango

asparagus

eggplant

watermelon

sweet potatoes

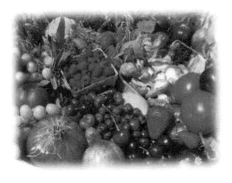

Why are some types of produce more prone to absorbing pesticides than others? Pineapple and sweet corn, for example, have a protective barrier in their outer layer of skin. Strawberries and lettuce do not.

The President's Cancer Panel recommends washing conventionally grown produce to remove residues. Researchers, however, say that while washing won't hurt and may help, it is impossible to eliminate all residues.

The lists of "dirty" and "clean" produce were compiled after the USDA washed the produce using high-power pressure water systems that most of us could only dream of having in our kitchens.

The full list contains 49 types of produce rated on a scale from least to most contaminated. You can check out the complete list at www.foodnews.org.

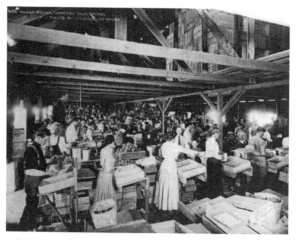

OHS Image bb012659- Commercial peach packing c. 1905; Thompson Fruit Company.

Broccoli For Just About Everything

The whole Brassica family contains key ingredients for fighting cancer. How these ingredients work is still largely a mystery. Researchers have learned that there are over 2,000 different nutrients and co-factors in any one food; they can identify about 200. All of these agents interact with human genes, turning gene response and expression on and off.

"Almost all aspects of life are engineered at the molecular level, and without understanding molecules we can only have a very sketchy understanding of life itself," said Francis Crick, PhD, co-discoverer of the DNA double helix.

"An increasing body of evidence has demonstrated that individual compounds —as well as complex mixtures of chemicals—derived from food alter the expression of genes in the human body. ... Studies based on ethnopharmacology and phytotherapy concepts showed that nutrients and botanicals can interact with the genome causing marked changes in gene expression."[67]

Broccoli is a green cruciferous vegetable and a member of the *italic cultivar* group. There are two main types of broccoli, heading and sprouting. Broccoli has been around for over 2,000 years and was first seen in Turkey. The Italian immigrants of the early 19th century carried broccoli to North America. It took another century for broccoli to become popular outside the Italian communities and develop into a commercial crop. Ninety percent of the broccoli grown in the United States comes from the Salinas Valley in California. During the winter months, Arizona, Texas, Florida and Washington take over production.

So Why Should You Eat Broccoli?

Mother always said to eat your broccoli, and she was right. Broccoli contains vitamins B1, B2, A, C, E and K, folic acid, calcium, chromium, indoles, isothiocynates (heavy duty cancer fighters) and sulforaphane glucosinolate. The best means of obtaining the health benefits of broccoli is to consume it fresh on a regular basis. A handful of three-day-old sprouts contains 50 times the sulforaphane glucosinolate as 114 pounds of regular broccoli. For those utilizing broccoli as a cancer-preventive food, I'd go with broccoli sprouts in my juice or salads every day. Bladder cancer is the 7th most common cancer worldwide, accounting for 3.2% of all cancers. In 2000 there were an estimated 260,000 new cases in men and 76,000 cases in women *(Ferlay et al., 2001).*

Benefits of Broccoli

- ✓ Cancer preventive (breast, bladder, stomach, colon and prostate cancer)
- ✓ Antioxidant (prevention of ophthalmic disorders/AMDR, anti-aging)
- ✓ Anti-inflammatory (prevention of cardiovascular disease, lowers LDL cholesterol, lowers blood pressure, helps prevent headaches and cramps, repairs damaged gastrointestinal mucosa)
- ✓ Enhances detoxification of heavy metals (arsenic), endogenous estrogens and xenoestrogens
- ✓ Neuro-protective (Parkinson's disease, Alzheimer's disease)
- ✓ Antibiotic (kills *helicobacter pylori*, sinus problems, herpes outbreaks, due to the indol-3-carbonal)

---

[67] (Phenolics, inflammation and nutrigenomics" J Sci Food Agric, 2006, Vol 86(15): 2503-1509)

A clinical trial in one of China's most polluted regions involving nearly 300 Chinese men and women found daily consumption of a half cup of broccoli sprout juice produced significant and sustained excretion of benzene, a known human carcinogen, and acrolein, a lung irritant. Johns Hopkins Bloomberg School of Public Health researchers, working with colleagues in the U.S. and China, used a plant compound called sulforaphane that had already demonstrated cancer preventative properties in animal studies.[68]

The way you prepare and consume your broccoli matters, according to a study from the University of Illinois. The study provides convincing evidence and also suggests steaming broccoli with broccoli sprouts may make the vegetable's anti-cancer effect almost twice as powerful.

"Broccoli, prepared correctly, is an extremely potent cancer-fighting agent—three to five servings a week are enough to have an effect. To get broccoli's benefits, though, the enzyme myrosinase has to be present; if it's not there, sulforaphane, broccoli's cancer-preventive and anti-inflammatory component, doesn't form," said Elizabeth Jeffery, a Univeristy of Illinois professor of nutrition.[69]

Remember to buy from a reputable local farm, farmer's market or from the organic section at your favorite grocery store. The best way to cook broccoli is to slightly steam it; this increases broccoli's cancer-fighting properties. Steam until it is tender but still crisp and bright green in color. You can also stir fry or wrap it in foil with other vegetables like peppers, tomatoes, onions and garlic. Add a pinch of thyme, basil and oregano and place on your grill to steam in its natural juices, and enjoy with your chicken or steak.

---

[68] Johns Hopkins Bloomberg School of Public Health. "Broccoli sprout beverage enhances detoxification of air pollutants in clinical trial." ScienceDaily. ScienceDaily, 16 June 2014. <www.sciencedaily.com/releases/2014/06/140616102410.htm>.
[69] University of Illinois College of Agricultural, Consumer and Environmental Sciences. "Sprouts? Supplements? Team them up to boost broccoli's cancer-fighting power." ScienceDaily. ScienceDaily, 31 January 2011. <www.sciencedaily.com/releases/2011/01/110127110707.htm>.

Place up to one cup of broccoli seeds into a clear glass jar and cover with water. Sprouting Jar's with a stainless steel screen and lid can be found in natural health food stores or from NOW®.

Alternatively, place broccoli seeds into a moist linen or muslin bag. Rinse or spray the broccoli seeds two to four times per day. Once rootlets and two leaves have formed, the seeds have become broccoli sprouts.

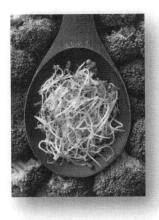

When fall approaches, my thoughts turn to warm and savory foods like onions. The thickness of the onion skin has been used to predict how severe the next winter may be; thin skins mean a mild winter and thick skins indicate a rough winter ahead. Onions, along with garlic, chives, shallots, leeks and green onions (scallions), are in the *Amaryllis* family—often incorrectly referred to as the Lily family. There are two basic types: the bulb forming favorites like Walla Walla, Vidalia and Spanish red onions and the perennials that produce clusters of onions that can be replanted. Cluster onions include shallots, Egyptian onions and garlic. This family of vegetables is cultivated worldwide and has been used for health as well as culinary purposes for millennia.

Onions originated in Central Asia—from Iran to Pakistan and northward to the Slavic countries. Onion gardens have been excavated that date back 5,000 years; Pharaohs were buried with onions to symbolize immortality. Documents dating back to the 6th century show onions being used medicinally in India. The Romans believed that onions could cure almost any ailment. Even though the onion itself was not spicy enough for the Greeks and Romans, they were heavily used for their pungency and were widely available to the poorer populations throughout the world.

Christopher Columbus and other explorers brought onions to the Americas. The three top vegetables of European cuisine from the Middle Ages to present are beans, cabbage and onions. Onions have been used as currency and given as wedding gifts.

Wild onions have been growing in North America since well before the Pilgrims' arrival. The Native Americans used wild onions for cooking, as seasoning in syrups and for dyeing textiles. Official onion cultivation began in America in 1629 and is now one of the top ten vegetable crops grown in the United States. The world's leading producers of onions are China, India, the United States, Turkey and Pakistan. In the United States, Idaho, Oregon, Washington, California and Texas are the largest producers.

Vitamin C, fiber, biotin, folate, chromium, vitamin K and thiamin are found in members of the onion family along with potent anti-cancer phytochemicals like quercetin, phenolic acid, sterols, pectin, volatile oils, sulfur compounds and the enzyme *alliinase*. It is this enzyme's release and its conversion to trans-S-cystine that causes the cook's eyes to water.

While not quite as highly valued medicinally as garlic, onions are widely used for similar purposes because they possess the same properties. Studies have shown that onion extracts, like those of garlic, decrease blood sugar and lipid levels, prevent clots, lower blood pressure, reduce inflammation (onions are one of the only foods that contain prostaglandin E1), improve asthma and allergies and retard viruses by improving the immune system. The blood sugar-lowering effects of onions have been clinically found to be comparable to that of prescription drugs *tolbutamide* and *phenformin*, commonly given to type 2 diabetics. Onions have been found to help the liver process glucose more efficiently by increasing the availability and natural secretion of insulin.

Historically, onions have been used in the treatment of asthma due to their ability to inhibit the production of compounds that cause bronchial spasms and mucous production. Onion extracts have been found to inhibit the formation of tumor cells and shallots exhibit significant activity against leukemia.

Health Benefits Of Onions

- Helps prevent cancer of the lung, breast, ovaries, kidney, prostate, skin, mouth, esophageal, stomach, colon and liver
- Helps prevent and treat diabetes, hypoglycemia, metabolic syndrome and insulin resistance
- Helps lower cholesterol and reduces the risk of atherosclerosis, cardiovascular disease, heart attack and stroke
- Helps to increase bone density and possibly decreases the risk of osteoporosis

Onions are available in fresh, frozen, canned and dehydrated forms; my preference is fresh as this form has the most nutritional benefits. Store your onions in a cool (55 degrees), dry location; this will help them retain their vitamin C content for as long as six months.

Onions are prone to contamination by *aflatoxin*, produced from *aspergillus parasiticus*, if incorrectly stored. Onions are often subjected to food irradiation in order to inhibit their sprouting potential; food irradiation can have various toxic effects. Onions may cause food allergies and trigger migraines in some people.

No matter how you fix them, onions are just plain good for you and they are a food that your cells know what to do with.

In my home we had canned and pickled sugar beets with a side of greens. For me, the beet greens were (and sometimes still are) the only edible part of the plant, but there are many people who love beets in all their forms.

Like many modern vegetables, beetroot was first cultivated by the Romans. In the 19th century it gained significant commercial value when it was discovered that beets could be converted into sugar. The Amalgamated Sugar Company was founded in 1897 in Logan, Utah, and is now located in Boise, Idaho. The company markets its sugar under the White Satin brand.

By the 1950s, White Satin sugar was in every grocery store in the Pacific Northwest. The company was listed on the New York Stock Exchange in 1950. A new distribution center in Portland, Oregon, was finished in 1951. The distribution silo could hold 2,500 tons of sugar and supply it as bulk, liquid, blended or packaged sugar. Classic beetroot recipes, such as borscht, are associated with central and Eastern Europe. Beets are in the same family as chard and spinach, and both the leaves and root can be eaten. The leaves have a bitter taste whereas the round root is sweet. Beets come in a variety of colors, including white and a creamy yellow. Beets can be eaten raw, cooked or pickled.

Beets are exceptionally healthy, especially the greens, which are rich in calcium, iron and vitamins A and C. Beetroots are an excellent source of folic acid and a splendid source of fiber, manganese and potassium. Beets help the liver to detoxify harmful chemicals from the body. The greens can be cooked up and enjoyed in the same way as spinach.

A unique source of phytonutrients called *betalains* are found in beets. Betanin and vulgaxanthin are the two best-studied betalains found in beets, and both have been shown to provide antioxidant, anti-inflammatory and detoxification support. Betalain red-colored pigments are found in other foods like the stems of chard and rhubarb, but the peel and flesh of beets offer an unusually high concentration.

An estimated 10-15% of U.S. adults experience beeturia (a reddening of the urine) after consumption of beets in everyday amounts. While this phenomenon is not harmful, it may possibly indicate problems with iron metabolism. Individuals with iron deficiency, iron excess, or particular problems with iron metabolism are much more likely to experience beeturia than individuals with healthy iron metabolism.

The word "pumpkin" comes from the Greek word "pepon" or "big melon". Pumpkins are members of the melon family, along with cantaloupes and watermelon. Pumpkins that make good jack-o'-lanterns are not necessarily the best for pie-making. For pies, my personal favorites are Sweetmeat or Hubbard squashes. Pumpkins come in a variety of colors in addition to orange, such as white, blue and red.

Pumpkin seeds found in Mexico have been estimated to be at least 7,500 years old. The pumpkin was a mainstay of Native American culture; it was used for food and the shell was used for making mats and other products. The first pumpkin pie was made by early American settlers; they filled the hollowed-out pumpkin with honey, milk and spices and baked it.

The biggest producers of pumpkin are the United States, India, China and Mexico. The pumpkin capital of the world is reported to be in Morton, Illinois, the location of the Libby processing plant.

Pumpkins play a role in preventing cancer, diabetes, hypertension and asthma.

Turnips

The first vegetable carved for Halloween was not the pumpkin, however, but the turnip. The turnip is a member of the cruciferous family, which also includes broccoli and cabbage. Both the root and the greens are eaten; the greens are smaller and more tender than those of their bigger family member, collard greens. Rutabagas are a cross between turnips and kale.

Turnips were cultivated almost 4,000 years ago in Asia. The Greeks and Romans further cultivated turnips into several varieties. In the Middle Ages they were widely grown throughout Europe until potatoes became popular in the 18th century. In Scotland and Ireland, turnips were carved and placed at doorways on All Hollows' Eve to ward off evil spirits.

Early European settlers brought the turnip to America; they grew well in the south and became a favorite food in local cooking. The greens from the turnip became a mainstay in African-American households. This may be because the traditional West African diet utilized a wide variety of greens.

Although turnips are a starch, they provide only a third of the calories as an equal amount of potatoes. They are an excellent source of fiber, vitamin C, folic acid, pantothenic acid, thiamine, niacin, potassium, magnesium, riboflavin, vitamin E, manganese and copper. The greens have a higher concentration of nutrients than the root itself.

Like all members of the cruciferous family, turnips are excellent cancer fighters.

Mushrooms

Mushrooms are the fruit of fungi called mycelium which grow in the soil, wood or decaying matter. There are thousands of known varieties and still more to be found. Some of the most popular varieties are black trumpet, chanterelle, clown ear, lobster, morel, oyster, porcini, portabello, shiitake, truffle, white button and wood ear mushrooms. Mushrooms convey a fifth taste sense, called *unami* in Japanese, which translates as savory or meaty.

Not all edible mushrooms are used for cooking; many have been found to contain medicinal benefits and are sold as supplements, teas or herbs. Eastern cultures have used mushrooms for both food and medicine for thousands of years. Ancient Egyptians believed that eating mushrooms would make one live forever. France was one of the first countries renowned for the cultivation of fungi. After King Louis XIV's reign, mushrooms gained popularity in England; in the late 19th century, cultivated mushrooms came to the United States.

China accounts for 32% of worldwide mushroom production and the United States cultivates 16%.

Mushroom of the gods, Agaricus blazei Murill, is a type of Brazilian mushroom. It is now grown in large quantities in Japan. Agaricus blazei Murill may help to prevent and treat various types of cancer. It may inhibit the formation of new blood vessels that feed tumors, help to prevent liver cancer, enhance the function of NK lymphocytes and improve the ability of NK lymphocytes to destroy cancer cells. It also may help normalize liver function in hepatitis B patients.

Mushroom Sugar, trehalose, is a disaccharide comprised of two glucose molecules. It is 45% as sweet as sucrose. Mushroom sugar may alleviate Huntington's disease.

Dancing Mushroom (Maitake mushroom) is a type of Japanese mushroom. Maitake mushrooms may improve immune system function with the onset of AIDS and may also inhibit the HIV virus from killing helper T-cells by up to 97% in 50% of AIDS patients. Maitake mushrooms may help to prevent many types of bacterial and viral diseases. Maitake mushrooms may help to prevent and treat cancer of the breast, liver, lung and prostate. Maitake mushrooms are believed to be useful in the treatment of chronic fatigue syndrome (CFS). They also help to lower elevated blood sugar levels and elevated serum triglycerides and may support weight loss. They also facilitate the growth of bone marrow and may reduce blood pressure.

The Oyster mushroom is another type of Japanese mushroom. It is cream and gray in color, with fluted caps. The Oyster mushroom is valued in culinary circles where it is often used in salads to provide a soft meaty texture and delicate flavor. Oyster mushrooms may lower blood pressure, help to prevent and treat ulcerative colitis, improve kidney function, prevent and treat some forms of cancer, and stimulate cell death of prostate cancer cells.

There are thousands of research articles, herbal citations and folk remedies that attest to the healing properties of mushrooms.

Potatoes: Red, White, Purple & Brown

The potato has a long history that started long before it accidentally washed up on the beaches of Ireland. Potatoes were cultivated for food for more than 2,000 years in South America. The Inca, it is believed, cultivated potatoes since 3000 B.C.

In the ancient ruins of Peru and Chile, archeologists have found potatoes dating back to 500 B.C. The Inca had many uses for potatoes, which varied in size from a small nut to an apple and in color from red and gold to blue and black. The Inca buried potatoes with their dead, stashed potatoes in concealed bins in case of war or famine and dried them and carried them on long journeys. They placed raw potato slices on broken bones, carried them to prevent rheumatism and ate them with other foods to prevent indigestion. The Inca also used potatoes to measure time by observing how long it took potatoes to grow.

Spanish explorer Gonzalo Jiminez de Quesada (1499-1579) took the potato to Spain in lieu of gold. "The Spanish believed the potato to be a type of truffle and called them 'tartuffo'. Potatoes were used on Spanish ships to prevent scurvy; this is due to the high vitamin C content of potatoes, and it was noted the sailors who ate potatoes did not suffer from scurvy.

"By 1585, the potato traveled to Italy and England, by 1587 to Belgium and Germany, to Austria in 1588 and to France around 1600. Wherever the potato was introduced, it was considered odd, poisonous or evil. In France and England, the potato was believed the cause of leprosy, syphilis, narcosis, scrofula, early death, sterility, rampant sexuality and poor soil."

An Irish legend claims that when ships of the Spanish Armada wrecked off the Irish coast in 1588, the ships were carrying potatoes that washed ashore. Other historical accounts report that Sir Walter Raleigh first brought the potato to Ireland and planted them at his Irish estate at Myrtle Grove, Youghal, near Cork, Ireland. Legend has it that he made a gift of the potato plant to Queen Elizabeth I. The local gentry were invited to a banquet featuring the potato in every course. Unfortunately, the cooks had no clue what to do with the potatoes and tossed out the lumpy-looking tubers. They instead brought to the royal table a dish of boiled stems and leaves (which are poisonous), and promptly made everyone deathly ill. The potatoes were then banned from court.

Antoine-Augustin Parmentier, a French military chemist and botanist, searching for a food to reduce famine, persuaded the king of France to let him plant 100 useless acres outside Paris, France, with potatoes. He asked the king to place troops around the fields to increase the interest of the local farmers. When the crop was ready for harvest, the troops were allowed the night off; the local farmers, as hoped, stole the potatoes and planted them. This was the beginning of potato farming, even if they were largely used as hog food for many years.

The "Great Famine" or "Great Starvation" in Ireland resulted from potato blights, a fungal infection in the soil. A book written in 1962 called *The Great Hunger: Ireland 1845-1849* by Cecil Woodham-Smith reads: "That cooking any food other than a potato had become a lost art. Women hardly boiled anything but potatoes. The oven had become unknown after the introduction of the potato prior to the Great Starvation."

Although potatoes are grown throughout the United States, no state is more associated with the potato than Idaho. In the 1850s, most Americans considered the potato food for animals rather than for humans. As late as the middle of the 19th century, the *Farmer's Manual* recommended that potatoes "be grown near the hog pens as a convenience towards feeding the hogs." It was not until the Russet Burbank potato was developed by American horticulturist Luther Burbank in 1872 that the Idaho potato industry really took off.

In the 1943-1947 *USDA Science in Farming Yearbook,* a whole chapter was dedicated to potato storage. "The storage of table stock potatoes also has become more complex. Potatoes for early consumption can be kept in warm-temperature storage with minimal air circulation, and it is now known that a higher vitamin content is retained by this treatment." [70] So those old-fashioned root cellars that were already in use really did affect the quality of the food.

Today, the potato is the most consumed vegetable in America. Because of its high glycemic rating and the addition of fat used in frying, this food has increased America's waistline considerably. We seem to forget that the potato has only been consumed by northern Europeans for a few hundred years and as such their DNA structure is not fully adapted to utilizing this starchy food. I personally love potatoes, but know I can only eat them in small quantities if I expect to dodge type 2 diabetes and heart disease.

Chocolate

Chocolate connoisseurs know there is more than gustatory pleasure to be found in this "food of the gods." In 1753, Carl von Linnaeus, a Swedish scientist, thought cacao was so important he named the genus and species of tree *Theobroma cacao* which literally means "cacao, the food of the gods."

Raw cacao, or theobroma cacao, is the seed in the fruit of the cacao tree. The food dated back to prehistoric times and was extensively cultivated in Mexico, Central and South America for years before the arrival of Europeans. [71]

The indigenous populations ate only the fruit, which offers many health benefits. The seed or cacao nib was reserved for their psychedelic brew, called *ayahuasca*, and for medicines. The Mayan Indians began cultivating cacao about 600 AD. According to Aztec myth, the cacao awakened power and wisdom. When the explorer Cortes brought cacao back with him upon returning to Spain in 1528, it was sequestered away and enjoyed only by the wealthy and nobility.

In medieval times and today, chocolate was and is seen as a luxury item and an indulgence, used as gifts for mothers and sweethearts. It is made into cocktails, cold and hot drinks, candies, powders, wines and lotions. The Spanish are widely responsible for the introduction and development of chocolate foods and drinks.

Cocoa naturally has a very strong, pungent taste, which comes from the flavonols. When cocoa is processed into your favorite chocolate products, it goes through several steps to reduce this taste. The more chocolate is processed (through fermentation, alkalizing, roasting, etc.), the more flavanols are lost. Most commercial

---

[70] The Yearbook of Agriculture 1943-1947 – Science in Farming, USDA, by Alfred D. Edgar page 871
[71] (Orey, 2010)

chocolates are highly processed. Flavonoids are naturally-occurring compounds found in plant-based foods that offer certain health benefits. They are part of the polyphenol group (chemicals found in plants). There are more than 4,000 flavonoid compounds, which are found in a wide variety of foods and beverages, such as cranberries, apples, peanuts, chocolate, onions, tea and red wine. Flavanols are a type of flavonoid specifically found in cocoa and chocolate.

Dark chocolate contains a large number of antioxidants (nearly eight times the amount found in strawberries). Flavonoids also help lower blood pressure through the production of nitric oxide; it can also balance certain hormones in the body. The fats in chocolate (1/3 oleic acid, 1/3 stearic acid and 1/3 palmitic acid) do not impact your cholesterol.

Dark chocolate helps restore flexibility to arteries while also preventing white blood cells from sticking to the walls of blood vessels. Both arterial stiffness and white blood cell adhesion are known factors that play a significant role in atherosclerosis. Scientists found that increasing the flavanol content of dark chocolate did not change this effect. This discovery was published in the March 2014 issue of *The FASEB Journal*.

"The effect that dark chocolate has on our bodies is encouraging not only because it allows us to indulge with less guilt, but also because it could lead the way to therapies that do the same thing as dark chocolate but with better and more consistent results," said Gerald Weissmann, MD, editor-in-chief of *The FASEB Journal*. "Until the 'dark chocolate drug' is developed, however, we'll just have to make do with what nature has given us!" [72]

Benefits Of Dark Chocolate

- ✓ Oleic acid is a healthy monounsaturated fat that is also found in olive oil
- ✓ Stearic acid is a saturated fat but one which research shows has a neutral effect on cholesterol
- ✓ Palmitic acid is also a saturated fat, one which raises cholesterol and heart disease risk (this is still under debate)
- ✓ Lowers blood pressure: Studies have shown that consuming a small bar of dark chocolate every day can reduce blood pressure
- ✓ Lowers cholesterol: Dark chocolate has been shown to reduce LDL cholesterol (the bad cholesterol) by up to 10 percent
- ✓ Stimulates endorphin production, which gives a feeling of pleasure
- ✓ Contains serotonin, which acts as an anti-depressant

---

[72] (Based on materials provided by Federation of American Societies for Experimental Biology.)

✓ Source of theobromine, caffeine and other substances which are stimulants

Chocolate is still a high-calorie, high-fat food. Most of the studies done used no more than 100 grams, or about 3.5 ounces, of dark chocolate a day. One bar of dark chocolate has around 400 calories. If you eat half a bar of chocolate a day, you must balance those 200 calories by eating less of something else. Cut out other sweets or snacks and replace them with chocolate to keep your total caloric consumption equal. Chocolate is a complex food with over 300 compounds and chemicals in each bite. Look for pure dark chocolate or dark chocolate with nuts, orange peel or other natural flavorings. To really enjoy and appreciate chocolate, take the time to taste it.

Enjoy moderate portions of chocolate (e.g., one ounce) a few times per week, and don't forget to consume other flavonoid-rich foods like apples, red wine, tea, onions and cranberries. Your best choices are dark chocolate instead of milk chocolate (especially milk chocolate that is loaded with other fats and sugars), and cocoa powder that has not undergone Dutch processing (cocoa that is treated with an alkali to neutralize its natural acidity).

Coffee: Black, If You Please

After oil, coffee is the second most traded commodity in the world. Coffee comes from an evergreen tree that produces red cherries, or beans. Most coffee comes from Arabica or Robusta varieties of beans. Arabica beans comprise 70% of the world's coffee production. Robusta coffee comes from southeast Asia and Brazil, contains about 50% more caffeine than Arabica and has a stronger, more bitter taste.

Africans fueled up on protein-rich coffee-and-animal-fat balls—primitive PowerBars®—and unwound with wine made from coffee berry pulp. Coffee traveled across the Red Sea to Arabia, where roasted beans were brewed around 1000 AD. By the 13th century Muslims were drinking coffee religiously. The "bean broth" powered dervishes, kept worshippers from falling asleep during prayers, and was part of daily life. Wherever Islam went, coffee went also—from North Africa to the eastern Mediterranean to India.[73, 74]

Arabia made beans infertile by parching or boiling them before exporting, and it is said that no coffee seed sprouted outside Africa or Arabia until the 1600s, when an

---

[73] Cortes, the Secret History of Coffee, Cocca & Cola
[74] http://www.serdas.com/coffee-history/

Indian pilgrim-cum-smuggler left Mecca with fertile seeds strapped to his belly. A merchant of Venice introduced Europe to coffee in 1615. The Dutch were the first to successfully transport a coffee plant into Europe in 1616. In 1696 they founded the first European-owned coffee estates in colonial Java, now part of Indonesia. Coffee came to the new world in 1727. Brazil's government wanted a chunk of the coffee market and used a spy to smuggle seeds from a coffee country. "Lt. Col. Francisco de Melo Palheta accomplished the task and is cited as the James Bond of Beans by National Geographic®."

In French Guiana, ostensibly to mediate a border dispute, emissary Palheta chose a path of pleasant resistance—the governor's wife. At a state farewell dinner she presented him a sly token of affection: a bouquet spiked with seedlings. By the 1800s, Brazil's monster harvests would turn coffee from an elite indulgence into a drink for the people.

Moderate intake of coffee is about three 6 ounce cups per day, for a total of 18 ounces daily. Coffee doesn't contain any significant amounts of vitamins or minerals, but it does contain antioxidants that rate higher than most other foods. An average cup of coffee contains between 60 and 130 mg of caffeine. Coffee is a stimulant, as are soda pops and energy drinks. Stimulants affect the brain and central nervous system, which can be both a good thing and a bad, depending on the situation and extent. Asthmatics may find they can breathe better and headache sufferers can speed the relief provided by aspirin by taking it with coffee or black tea. Coffee consumption has been found to be beneficial for reducing inflammation and preventing heart disease in non-caffeine sensitive postmenopausal women. One study also found that elderly men had less memory loss when consuming three cups of coffee daily. The University of Arizona found that drinking decaffeinated coffee had the reverse effect.

On the other hand, coffee consumption can increase fibrocystic breast disease, hypertension, dehydration, sleep disturbances and acid indigestion. Added artificial flavorings, cream and sugar can increase asthma restriction, raise blood sugars and cause weight gain by increasing stress hormones and adding calories. If these added flavors are the only way you can drink coffee, find a better way to wake up—one that helps your brain work better, not jitterier.

Remember that coffee is a burden to your kidneys. For every cup of coffee you drink, your kidneys need one quart of water to flush and prevent kidney stone formation. As with everything, enjoy that cup (6-12 oz) of coffee in moderation. Select high-quality, fragrant, organic brands and go easy on the artificial flavors and refined sugars.

Fermentation is making a big comeback. Artisan bread makers are developing their own strains of yeast, kombucha makers are popping bottles of fizzy drinks at farmers' markets and online gurus are creating websites dedicated to specialty fermenting jars and gadgets. I have clients swapping kimchee and sauerkraut recipes like we used to do with the "banana bread sourdough starter" in years past. (I'm not sure if anyone ever made the banana bread—I think we just kept passing the jar of starter around hoping it would not swallow us in our sleep.)

Health-wise, sourdough and other fermented products are great ways to reintroduce natural probiotics back into the digestive system. This is the traditional, economical way of preventing many illnesses related to digestion. Every culture has some form of fermented food that is consumed almost daily. Here is one Finnish fermented food shared by a client who lives in Washington.

Finnish Sima Spring Mead

A lightly fermented lemonade. If you drink this sparkling beverage as soon as the raisins float, it's fine to serve to the kids as well! But be warned—Sima transforms from being slightly bubbly to being very bubbly and slightly intoxicating the longer that it ferments.

Ingredients
1 1/4 gallon water (5 liters)
2 lemons
1/2 cup brown sugar
1/2 cup white sugar plus sugar for the bottles
1/4 tsp dry yeast
25 raisins

Peel lemons with a potato peeler, taking off just the rind. Remove the white pulp layer and toss it. Slice lemon and rind. Place lemon and sugar into a large, NON-METAL, bowl. Bring the water to a boil and pour boiling water over the lemons and sugar. Let the mixture cool until lukewarm. Dissolve the yeast in lukewarm water for a few minutes. Add it to the lukewarm mixture. Stir it briefly.

Let the mixture ferment at room temperature overnight. (I covered mine with a lid.) Pour through a sieve and then bottle it. Put 4-5 raisins and a teaspoon of sugar into each bottle before closing. Keep bottles at room temperature for a few hours, and then store upright in a cool place like a pantry for a couple of days. Then put it in the refrigerator and store it there. The drink is ready to serve in a few days, but is best in a week. Raisins float to top when it's ready to taste.

The earlier you use it the more you can taste the lemon. We like it at least seven days old—it becomes clear and more like a cider. Be sure to open over the sink if you hold it that long because it can come out of the bottle like champagne. Use glass bottles, please.

Yogurt

Years ago, my dad gave me a food dehydrator as a gift. One of the reasons I wanted a dehydrator was so I could make my own yogurt. I had been introduced to this tangy dairy food by my mother-in-law. The version she made was so tart it gave lemons a run for their money and I was sure I could make it more palatable. I did, too. But as the years passed, I, like millions of others, began to rely on store brands for my yogurt and kefir.

Dairy allergies are far more widespread and more complex than the term "lactose intolerance" implies. Lactose is only one component of dairy that can irritate the digestive lining and create mucous. Excess mucus can clog up sinus passages and lung airways, cause constipation and interfere with the gut's ability to absorb nutrients.

The popular press, TV ads and medical journals are awash with information on the healing benefits of probiotics; they claim that one can lose unwanted weight by eating yogurt, as if it were only that simple. The problem is that most of the commercial foods available, like Activa™ and Dannon™ products, are pretty much dead. Studies have shown that the majority of "active" cultures in 98% of the grocery store yogurts are useless for repopulating the gut. They also found that it was actually the sucralose and other additives like propylene glycol and inulin that boosted bowel regularity in consumers.

Take a look at all the additives in one popular "natural" brand:

So Delicious™ Cultured Coconut Milk ingredients: organic coconut milk (water, organic coconut cream), chicory root extract, pectin, algin, magnesium phosphate, tricalcium phosphate, rice starch, locust bean gum, live cultures, guar gum, dipotassium phosphate, gellan gum, xanthan gum, vitamin d2, vitamin b12.

So Delicious™ Blueberry Greek Cultured Coconut Milk ingredients: organic coconut milk (water, organic coconut cream), chicory root extract, blueberries, organic dried cane syrup, rice starch, pectin, tapioca dextrose, natural flavor, algin (kelp extract), magnesium phosphate, tricalcium phosphate, blueberry juice concentrate, locust bean gum, live cultures, citric acid, grape, carrot and blueberry juices for color, guar gum, monk fruit extract, sodium citrate, vitamin d-2, vitamin b12.

After discovering this I thought, why not make my own dairy-free fermented foods? After all, if SO™ and other companies can do it, so can I. Thanks to the information available on the Internet, it wasn't hard to find out how to make my own coconut milk yogurt. No more feeling deprived over the loss of another favorite food due to food sensitivities driving inflammation (a pounding sinus headache can be the result of inflammation caused by a food driving up your prostaglandin 2 production).

Coconut Milk Yogurt
2 cans organic coconut milk (carrageenan free)
2 probiotic nutritional supplement capsules
1 tsp real vanilla extract (optional)
3 Tbsp organic honey (optional)
3-4 Tbsp organic coconut oil (optional for added thickness if looking for a Greek yogurt)
1 glass quart jar

Instructions

1. Blend coconut milk with contents of probiotic capsules. Transfer to a 1 quart glass jar with a tight-fitting lid. (If you have an immersion blender, just dump everything into the jar and blend it right there.)

2. Store somewhere warm in your house, like on a window sill. After 24-48 hours, it should smell yogurt-y. It may be runny, more like kefir than yogurt. If you prefer, leave it out longer. After 48-72 hours, it should be thick and have a more tangy flavor.

3. Store in the refrigerator for up to 7 days.

4. Add fresh or frozen berries or homemade jams for flavors

Yogurt adds zest to salads, smoothies, granola and other foods. If you are Scandinavian, congratulations on reconnecting with an important aspect of you food history. It was the Scandinavians who invented many of these healthy fermented dairy foods.

Bread is older than metal. Even before the Bronze Age, our ancestors were eating and baking flat breads. There is evidence of neolithic grinding stones used to process grains. The oldest bread yet found is a loaf discovered in Switzerland, dating from 3500 BC.

Since California's gold mining days, sourdough has been a Western staple, delighting generations with its tangy flavor in breads, pancakes and other baked foods. This style of baking goes back to the ancient Egyptians, and Europeans have baked with sourdough starters for centuries. There is some discussion about how this process happened, and the degree to which there was an overlap between brewing and bread-making. Until the time of the development of commercial yeasts, all leavened bread was made using naturally occurring yeasts (i.e. all bread was sourdough, with its slower raise). One of the reasons given for the importance of unleavened bread in the Jewish faith is that at the time of the Exodus from Egypt, there wasn't time to let the dough rise overnight.

From Egypt, bread-making spread north to ancient Greece where it was a luxury product first produced in the home by women and later in commercial bakeries. The Greeks enjoyed over 70 different types of bread, including both savory and sweetened loaves, using a number of varieties of grain. The Romans learned the art of bread-making from the Greeks and made improvements on kneading and baking techniques. There are sourdough recipes dating from 17th century France using a starter which is fed and risen three times before adding it to the dough. The French were obviously far more interested in a good-tasting bread than they were in providing a comfortable life for the baker.

The introduction of commercial yeasts in the 19th century placed speed and consistency of production over taste and quality. By 1910, government regulations preventing night work and restricting working hours made more labor-intensive production less sustainable. In response, bakers favored faster-rising breads, such as the baguette.

In Germany, the use of sourdough was universal until brewers' yeasts became common in the 15th and 16th centuries. The overlap between brewing and baking was reflected in monasteries producing both bread and beer, using the heat of the oven to dry malted grain and the yeast to raise the bread. However, the big difference was that in Germany, sourdoughs continued to be used for rye breads, even as bakers' yeasts became more popular for all other types.

While yeast is still used with rye flours, the sourdough is used to increase acidity, which prevents starches from degrading. This use in Germany is also seen in other countries with a strong rye bread tradition such as the Scandinavian countries and the Baltic states. One great advantage of sourdough is you don't need to buy yeast. Having a way to make bread, in the rough and tumble world of mining and exploring, attracted the use of prospectors and explorers in the United States in the 19th century; the prospectors themselves were referred to as sourdoughs, and they would lend their name to the "mother" for growing yeast in for making bread. According to some reports, it was a practice to keep your mother leavening on your person, to make sure it didn't freeze in the bitter winters in mining areas in Alaska, Montana, Nevada and Idaho.

"Wild yeast and bacteria in the flour, liquid, and the air break down natural sugars and produce carbon dioxide, which enables bread baked with sourdough starter to rise. As it ferments, the starter provides acidity—in the form of lactic acid and some acetic acid—creating the 'sour' in sourdough. Once established, a starter can be kept for decades. Boudin Bakery, founded in San Francisco in 1849 and still operating, traces its sourdough starter to one begun more than 150 years ago by Isidore Boudin."[75, 76]

Some schools of thought assert naturally fermented foods can improve the digestive health of those with gluten sensitivities. However, I suggest sticking to gluten-free sourdough just to be on the safe side; after all, your health is worth the challenge. Here is a sourdough starter recipe from King Arthur Flour Company.[77]

GF Sourdough Starter
Add zest to your gluten-free breads and baked goods with this sourdough starter from King Arthur Mills.

Ingredients
1/4 tsp Florapan French Sourdough Starter or 1 package active yeast
1 cup Ancient Grains Flour Blend
1/2 cup lukewarm water
1 cup Gluten-Free Multi-Purpose Flour (Added on day 4 of the process)

---

[75] http://kitchenproject.com/history/sourdough.htm
[76] Food in History, Reay Tannahill
[77] www.kingarthurflour.com

Tips

- For a fun experiment, try substituting 1/2 cup starter for 1/2 cup of the flour and 2 ounces (1/4 cup) of the liquid in a gluten-free blueberry muffin recipe or any other muffin, cake or quick bread of your choice.
- For tangier yeast bread recipes, try using 1 cup starter in place of 1/2 cup water and 1 cup flour.
- Sourdough starter is best stored in the fridge in a stoneware crock or glass container with a loose-fitting lid.
- You should observe the same procedures for care and maintenance as for a wheat-based starter.

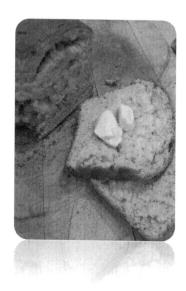

Healthy carbohydrates contain soluble and insoluble fibers. Fiber is our housekeeping team; not only does it keep our bowels moving , thereby reducing the risk factors for colon cancer, it also removes toxins and lowers blood sugars, blood pressure and cholesterol.

Consumers in the United States spend roughly $30 billion annually total on weight loss and an estimated $1-2 billion on weight loss programs. Research has proven that reducing the amount of calories you consume, managing stress and becoming more active is the only way to lose weight and maintain your ideal body weight What is not often discussed, however, is nature's built-in environmental protection agent, fiber.

By definition, fiber is the indigestible part of fruits, vegetables, seeds, whole grains and herbs.[78] Fiber and fiber-rich foods are natural regulators and an efficient clean-up crew removing toxins, congestion, unneeded fats and sugar. This reduces inflammation, a primary contributor to chronic illness.[79]

America's escalating cancer, diabetes, heart disease and obesity rates are a reflection of a country consuming a high-calorie diet devoid of fiber. Cake or carrots? Timing may decide what you'll eat and how much fiber you're getting. "In typical food choices, individuals need to consider attributes like health and taste in their decisions," says graduate student Nicolette Sullivan, lead author of the study, which appears in the December 15, 2014 issue of the journal *Psychological Science*. "What we wanted to find out was at what point the taste of the foods starts to become integrated into the choice process, and at what point health is integrated."

There are so many widely varying opinions about nutrients like fats and fiber that it's hard to find a definitive answer. Researchers at California Institute of Technology assumed the healthiness of a food is not factored into a person's food choice until after taste is. And for those individuals who exercised less self-control, they hypothesized, health would factor into the choice even later.[80]

By consuming more soluble and insoluble forms of fiber through healthy food choices, you can improve the health of your entire body, from your brain to your

---

[78] (Tabers, 2001)
[79] (Brenda Watson, 2007)
[80] California Institute of Technology. "Cake or carrots? Timing may decide what you'll eat." ScienceDaily. ScienceDaily, 15 December 2014. <www.sciencedaily.com/releases/2014/12/141215154633.htm>.

bowels. Fiber is not thought of as a nutrient but it should be; especially when you look at the 15 ways fiber helps the human digestive system work:

- ✓ Lose weight and maintain weight
- ✓ Increase energy
- ✓ Reduce heart disease
- ✓ Lower or maintain healthy cholesterol levels
- ✓ Reduce diabetes risk and regulate blood sugars
- ✓ Reduce cancer risk
- ✓ Maintain bowel regularity
- ✓ Reduce diverticulitis
- ✓ Regulate IBS (irritable bowel syndrome)
- ✓ Reduce body odor; improve skin and hair
- ✓ Improve immune function
- ✓ Balance brain chemistry
- ✓ Reduce headaches and allergies
- ✓ Prevent GERD or stomach nausea associated with slow transit time (constipation)
- ✓ Detoxify the body of hormone-disrupting chemicals and environmental toxins [81]

The average American consumes 4-8 grams of fiber per day. The American Diabetic Association recommends as much as 40 grams of fiber per day and the RDA for fiber is 20 grams. Now, I may not agree with the RDA on many things, but this much is clear: Americans of all ages are not eating enough fiber-rich foods.

How do we go about getting more fiber in our diet?

Start by eating real foods like berries, cherries, apples and greens. Consider adding a natural fiber supplement to your daily program such as psyllium seed, acacia fiber, chia seeds or flax seed (add flax only if you are a female and not estrogen dominate). Skip the Metamucil as it's full of artificial dyes, flavors and chemicals and also costs more.

When you introduce fiber supplements, start with half the recommended dose for two weeks to give your gut time to adjust to the increase in fiber. If you develop gas, bloating or cramps, increase the amount of water you consume daily or change the type of fiber supplement. Other beverages do not have the same effect as water and

---

[81] (Brenda Watson, 2007)

can actually contribute to the symptoms by acting as diuretics and preventing your digestive system from getting an adequate fluid supply.

Fiber adds bulk to your meals and creates a sense of fullness; this naturally reduces your calorie consumption and slows down the eating process. This allows your digestive system, hormones and brain to take their time. Bowels are a soft muscle and just like every other muscle, require exercise to stay healthy. Fiber traps chemicals, fats, prescription medications, oil-soluble nutrients like omega 3, 6 and 9, water and undigested food particles as it moves through the small and large intestines. This is why fiber is so effective in reducing diarrhea for those with IBS, ulcerative colitis or ileostomies.

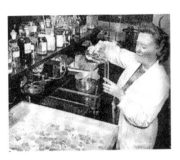

Image Right: A laboratory aide measures out the right amount of apple essence to give candy an apple flavor.

Lower Image: To study changes in freezing food at home, Equipment Specialist Dorothy Skinner inserts a thermocoupler into a carton of liquid.

Yearbook of Agriculture 1943-1947 Science in Farming

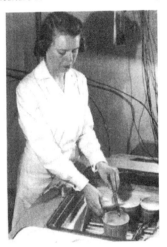

How do you know if your bowels are not "up to speed"? Take a transit time test. Eat an "indicator food" that will show up in your stool such as corn, beets, dark chocolate or sesame seeds. Then, time how long it takes from the time you eat the food until you see it in the toilet bowl. The ideal time ranges from 12 to 15 hours. Two to three bowel movements daily, if well-formed and easy (no straining or sprinting), are optimum.

The following list gives an idea of how much fiber you can add to your diet via everyday foods and supplements.

1 cup cooked black beans = 19.4 grams
3/4 cup lightly cooked broccoli = 7.0 grams
1/2 cup cooked spinach = 7.0 grams
1 cup red lentils = 6.4 grams
1 med yam cooked = 6.8 grams
3/4 cup Heritage™ heirloom whole grains organic cereal = 6 grams
1 cup whole grain spaghetti = 5.6 grams
1 tsp psyllium seed = 5 grams
1/4 cup uncooked quinoa = 5 grams
1 Tbsp golden flax seed meal = 5 grams
1 Cliff ™bars = 5 grams
1/2 cup raspberries = 4.6 grams
1/2 cup raw blackberries = 4.4 grams
1/2 cup cooked greens = 4.0 grams

Popcorn, The Fun Fiber

A Little History

Biblical accounts of "corn" stored in the pyramids of Egypt are actually a reference to other grains such as barley. The word "corn" was commonly used to refer to various grains in Europe such as wheat, barley and rye. In Scotland and Ireland, the term "corn" referred to oats. Maize was the ordinary American corn.

It is believed that the first use of wild and early cultivated corn was popping. Archeologists have found traces of popcorn in 1,000-year-old Peruvian tombs.[82] The oldest ears of popcorn ever found were discovered in the Bat Cave of west central New Mexico in 1948 and 1950. Ranging from smaller than a penny to about 2 inches, the oldest Bat Cave ears are about 4,000 years old.

Popcorn was integral to early 16th century Aztec Indian ceremonies. In 1519, Cortes got his first sight of popcorn when he invaded Mexico and came into contact with the Aztecs. Writing of Peruvian Indians in 1650, the Spaniard Cobo says, "They toast a certain kind of corn until it bursts. They call it pisancalla, and they use it as a confection."

The use of the moldboard plow became commonplace in the mid-1800s and led to the widespread planting of maize in the United States. Popcorn was very popular from the 1890s until the Great Depression. Street vendors used to follow crowds around, pushing steam or gas-powered poppers through fairs, parks, and expositions.

According to the Popcorn Board website, "Charles Cretors, founder of C. Cretors and Company in Chicago, introduced the world's first mobile popcorn machine at the World's Columbian Exposition in Chicago in 1893. Scientific American reported: 'This machine ... was designed with the idea of moving it about to any location where the operator would be likely to do a good business. The apparatus, which is light and strong, and weighing but 400 or 500 pounds, can be drawn readily by a boy or by a small pony to any picnic ground, fair, political rally, etc. and to many other places where a good business could be done for a day or two.'"

Popcorn at 5 or 10 cents a bag was one of the few luxuries down-and-out families could afford. During the Great Depression, the popcorn business thrived while other businesses failed. A slump did happen during the early 1950s, with the arrival of TV.

---

[82] http://www.history.com/news/hungry-history/a-history-of-popcorn

Attendance at movie theaters dropped and, with it, popcorn consumption. A new relationship between TV and popcorn was formed.

Many of us have fond memories of making Jiffy Pop™. Developed in 1958 by Frederick C. Mennen of LaPorte, Indiana, JiffyPop™ made it big when in the 1970s, the stage magician Henri Bouton fils, better known as Harry Blackstone, Jr., was endorsing the television commercial jingle called "the magic treat—as much fun to make as it is to eat." [83]

Did you know that microwave popcorn was the very first use of microwave heating in the 1940s? Percy Spencer, of Raytheon Manufacturing Corporation®, figured out how to mass produce magnetrons which were being used to generate microwaves for use in World War II. Looking for post-war applications of Raytheon technology, Spencer spurred the development of the microwave oven. Popcorn was key to many of Spencer's experiments.

The first patent for a microwave popcorn bag was issued to General Mills® in 1981, and home popcorn consumption increased by tens of thousands of pounds in the years following. Americans today consume 15 billion quarts of popped popcorn each year. The average American eats about 49 quarts.[84]

According to the non-GMO shopping guide, available for free at www.nongmoshoppingguide.com, there is no GMO popcorn, nor is there blue or red GM corn chips (although blue and red corn chips may have GM contamination).[85] Here are a few companies I like; however, I have not done a background check on these to see if they are secretly owned by ConAgra Foods®, Cargill® or Monsanto®. Even I can only handle so much before my mouth and tummy win out so I stick with local, reputable companies in my state, like Bob's Red Mill®.

I also like Boulder Canyon Natural Foods®, Glutino®, Edward & Sons®, Hail Merry®, Kettle Foods®, Tree of Life®, Lundberg Family Farms®, Arrowhead Mills®, Eden®, Great Northern® and NOW®.

Our family likes to sit in the yard on a summer night, hang a sheet on the shop wall and use the projector to screen movies while we enjoy our organic buttered popcorn. Just like the ol' fashioned drive-in, but better.

---

[83] http://www.history.com/news/hungry-history/a-history-of-popcorn
[84] http://www.popcorn.org
[85] www.nongmoshoppingguide.com

Fat

How is it that for centuries our ancestors consumed large quantities of high-fat foods and never fell victim to the health challenges of contemporary generations? To answer this, we must look at the lifestyle, food and preparation methods commonly used by past generations. The foods they consumed came from their own garden or local farms; they sometimes had periods of fasting or calorie reduction due to weather, income and harvest. The terms "processed" and "organic" were unheard of; everything from condiments to the main course were made from scratch.

Lifestyle and environmental factors have also dramatically changed over time. Every human in history must deal with some stress and trauma, but today we suffer from background stressors we may not even be fully aware of such as noise, electricity and artificial light. This in addition to our modern food preparation and farming practices contribute to the growing chronic health challenges we now face.

Many believe that people live much longer now than they used to; what has actually changed is childhood life expectancy. Because more infants and children survive to adulthood, the average reflects a longer life expectancy. In fact, Americans are only living on average 5 to 7 years longer than they did 100 years ago.

The next question is, do those years represent quality of life or just quantity? The American lifestyle has dramatically changed over the past century; we are now largely a sedentary society, consuming on average 900-2500 more calories daily than we can burn. Many now consume more plastic and petroleum byproducts than wholesome natural foods.

And just when did we begin to develop deficiencies in cholesterol-lowering medications? I'm convinced that an excess of highly processed synthetic fats and devitalized foods combined with a widespread misconception of the role of cholesterol has led to the overuse of cholesterol-lowering medications.[86, 87, 88]

Over the past few decades, the majority of Americans replaced so-called "bad" saturated fats from animal and plant sources of polyunsaturated fats like corn, cottonseed, sunflower and canola oil. All of these oils are from predominately GM crops, are loaded with chemicals and are processed at high temperatures with chemical solvents. These oils have been shown to elevate prostaglandin 2 markers which exacerbates inflammation and increases the risk of cancer.

---

[86] (Mary G. Enig, (2003)
[87] (University of California Dept. of Internal Medicine, 2010)
[88] Death by Food Pyramid (2013) Denise Minger

In every study I reviewed, these oils (initially) caused cholesterol levels to decrease while increasing markers for inflammation, diabetes, liver enzymes and cancer.

Fat is the generic term for fats (solid) and oils (liquid) in foods. All fats are triglycerides: mixtures of saturated, unsaturated and polyunsaturated fatty acids. Fatty acids are the building blocks of fat. They are described as saturated, unsaturated and polyunsaturated. Two of these fatty acids are required in the diet, making them essential fatty acids: *linolenic acid* and *alpha-linolenic acid*. These fats are most commonly found in cold water fish such as Alaskan salmon; free range grass-fed beef and poultry; wild game and high-quality omega-3 oil supplements. [89, 90]

Fat is necessary to add flavor and moisture to the diet. It is a key macronutrient, used for energy, brain function, hormones, nerve development, insulation and weight control. [91] For the past thirty years, Americans have been led to believe (by the media and those who have the most to gain financially), that fat is bad and that a diet high in carbohydrates is heart-healthy and better for you.

Instead, we have replaced healthy fats like coconut oil, olive oil and yes, real butter and eggs with highly processed fats that convert to prostaglandin 2 (found in polyunsaturated, hydrogenated omega-6 vegetable oils), an inflammation driver that leads to heart disease, high cholesterol, type 2 diabetes and inflammatory illnesses such as arthritis, gout, fibromyalgia and some believe, dementia. [92, 93, 94, 95]

No longer is it advisable to render your own fats from poultry, beef and pork, mostly due to the commercial use of large quantities of antibiotics, petroleum and hormone-disrupting chemicals which are stored by both animals and humans in body fat.

Humans are omnivores and are designed to consume real fats found in eggs, flesh and plant foods such as avocados, nuts, seeds, fruits, olives and coconut.

Fat provides energy and insulation and it slows down the conversion of carbohydrates like rice, corn, bread, sugar, dairy and potatoes to glucose (sugar). This gives the pancreas time to determine just how much insulin the body really needs. By keeping these two chemicals in check with healthy "real" fats,

---

[89] (Mary G. Enig, (2003)

[90] (Doyle, 2008)

[91] (Nestle, What to Eat, 2006)

[92] (Sci., 2010)

[93] (Centur, 2010)

[94] (Foundation, 2010)

[95] (O., 2006)

the human body is able to control inflammation, which is the root cause of degenerative illnesses like type 2 diabetes and heart disease.

In the past, fat has been considered the enemy of good nutrition, but when included in a healthy diet it boasts several potential health benefits. In the September 2014 issue of *Food Technology* magazine, published by the Institute of Food Technologists (IFT), Linda Milo Ohr wrote on how fatty acids and nutritional oils may benefit cognition, weight management, heart health, mood, and eye and brain development.

Here is a sample:

1. Omega-3 Fatty Acids: associated with brain development, cognition, eye health, dementia, heart health and depression.

2. Pinolenic Acid: based on pine nut oil derived from Korean pine tree, is rich in long-chain fatty acids, shown to suppress appetite and promote a feeling of fullness.

3. Conjugated Linoleic Acid: for weight management

4. Hemp Oil: contains a balanced ratio of omega-6 and omega-3 linolenic essential fatty acids, and also contains vitamin E.

5. Fish Oil: for its beneficial effect on cardiovascular, neurological and cognitive health.

6. Coconut Oil: aids in energy production, skin, and dental health.[96]

Olive Oil

Research has been accumulating on olive oil's health-protective properties. The phytonutrient components in olive oil are effective against breast cancer cells and studies suggest the abundance of olive oil in the Mediterranean way of eating may account for why the diet helps prevent depression. Now scientists have discovered that phenolic compounds in olive oil directly repress genes linked to inflammation.

A research team took blood samples after meals to check for the expression of over 15,000 human genes. The results? The high phenol olive oil clearly impacted the regulation of almost 100 genes, many of which have been linked to obesity, high blood fat levels, type 2 diabetes and heart disease.

---

[96] http://www.ift.org/food-technology/past-issues/2014/september/columns/nutraceuticals.aspx

"We identified 98 differentially expressed genes when comparing the intake of phenol-rich olive oil with low-phenol olive oil. Several of the repressed genes are known to be involved in pro-inflammatory processes, suggesting that the diet can switch the activity of immune system cells to a less deleterious inflammatory profile, as seen in metabolic syndrome," Dr. Perez-Jimenez said in a statement to the press. "These findings strengthen the relationship between inflammation, obesity and diet and provide evidence at the most basic level of healthy effects derived from virgin olive oil consumption in humans."

The ability of olive oil's phenolic compounds to reduce or prevent inflammation also provides a molecular basis for the reduction of heart disease observed in Mediterranean countries, where virgin olive oil represents a primary source of dietary fat.

This could be especially important in halting the dangerous effects of metabolic syndrome. Characterized by excess abdominal fat, high cholesterol, high blood pressure and high blood glucose levels, metabolic syndrome is linked to type 2 diabetes, heart disease and early death. [97]

But the next time you reach for a bottle of extra virgin olive oil, beware. A study from the University of California-Davis found more than two-thirds of imported extra virgin olive oil bottles are not what they seem. To be extra virgin, olive oil can't be rancid or doctored with lesser oils. The fruit must be the perfect size, color and ripeness. When UC-Davis's lab tested the most common 14 brands, they all failed one or more of the trials. "It's become a very sophisticated practice, the adulteration of olive oil throughout the world," Shoemaker says. The lab can prove defects, degradation and dilution in olive oil beyond what human taste buds can figure out. Often, olive oil is cut or blended with several other oils like hazelnut, soybean, sunflower and other types of oil.

There is no legal definition in the U.S. for grades of olive oil, but mounting concern over truth-in-olive-oil-labeling has drawn in the USDA. Since October 2010, regulations are conformed to international standards. Olive oil from every olive oil-producing country, including the U.S., is subject to random sampling off retail shelves.

There are health benefits to all natural oils when they are fresh and free from heavy metal contamination. So whether you are of Mediterranean descent or not,

---

[97] King's College London. "Why you need olive oil on your salad." ScienceDaily. ScienceDaily, 19 May 2014. <www.sciencedaily.com/releases/2014/05/140519160712.htm>.

take up the fun of olive oil tasting. There are companies like Temecula Oil Company, in California, that have a wonderful selection of oils and vinegars.

Over 60% of the brain is made up of cholesterol; all of our hormones are as well. Without healthy fats in our diet the liver is forced to make cholesterol to meet the body's needs for these essential components. There is a direct correlation with lower cholesterol and increases in depression, impaired immune function, muscle weakness and hormone imbalances.[98]

Many consumers believe that manufacturers' proclamations of "fat-free", "no trans-fats", "heart healthy" and "zero cholesterol" equal "good for you". The corn industry and the companies who profit off of it (McDonald's®, Coke®, Monsanto®, Cargill®, et al.) may be partly responsible for many of the modern health problems in America. The consumer must take their share of the blame also.

A local egg farmer on average receives .40 cents on every dollar of eggs sold. In contrast, a corn farmer only receives .02 cents on every dollar. According to Michael Pollan in his book *The Omnivore's Dilemma*, the bulk of the profit goes to big business like McDonald's® and Coca Cola®. High fructose corn sweetener, only one of the hundreds of products made from #2 corn, is the leading cause of non-alcoholic fatty liver disease, obesity and elevated cholesterols. Not the healthy fats found in real foods like organic butter, eggs, meats and fresh whole vegetables.[99]

It is my opinion and that of many others that cholesterol is one of the most unfairly maligned and unnecessarily "treated" naturally occurring blood components in the health industry today.

Coconut Oil

Now, I am about to get some health care providers' knickers in a knot. Those of you born in the 1940s or 1950s may remember a time when coconut oil and palm oil were in prepared foods. Then in the 1970s and 1980s we were told that these oils were bad for us and a leading cause of heart disease. Before we knew it, new "healthy oils" were in our favorite foods; canola and soybean oils had taken over the market almost overnight.

---

[98] (Mary G. Enig, (2003)
[99] (Pollan, The Omnivore's Dilemma, 2006)

Early Spanish explorers called the coconut "coco", which means "monkey face" because the three indentations (eyes) on the hairy nut resembles the head and face of a monkey. The coconut provides a nutritious source of meat, juice, milk and oil and it has fed and nourished populations around the world for generations.

Nearly one-third of the world's population depends on coconut to some degree for their food and their economy. In these cultures, the coconut has a long and respected history. Coconut is highly nutritious and rich in fiber, vitamins and minerals. It is classified as a "functional food" because it provides many health benefits beyond its nutritional content. [100, 101]

In traditional medicine around the world, coconut is used to treat a wide variety of health problems including abscesses, asthma, baldness, bronchitis, bruises, burns, colds, constipation, cough, dropsy, dysentery, earache, fever, flu, gingivitis, gonorrhea, irregular or painful menstruation, jaundice, kidney stones, lice, malnutrition, nausea, rash, scabies, scurvy, skin infections, sore throat, swelling, syphilis, toothache, tuberculosis, tumors, typhoid, ulcers, upset stomach, weakness and wounds.

Some of these treatments may not have any efficacy, but until the research is done, the jury is still out.

Modern Health Uses

Published studies in medical journals show that coconut, in one form or another, may provide a broad range of health benefits. Some of these are summarized below, however it is still unclear just how coconut oil kills many viruses and bacterium:

- Anti-parasitic, viral, bacterial and fungal
- Boosts energy and endurance
- Improves digestion and absorption of nutrients, and insulin secretion and utilization of blood glucose
- Reduces symptoms associated with pancreatitis
- Protect against osteoporosis
- Relieve symptoms associated with gallbladder disease, Crohn's disease, ulcerative colitis, and stomach ulcers
- Improves digestion and bowel function
- Relieves pain and irritation caused by hemorrhoids
- Anti-inflammatory
- Improves cholesterol ratio
- Helps prevent periodontal disease and tooth decay

---

[100] (Bruce Fife, Stop Alzheimer's Now!, 2011)
[101] (Bruce Fife, The Healing Miracles of Coconut Oil, 2003)

- A protective antioxidant. Does not deplete the body's antioxidant reserves like other oils do
- Relieve symptoms associated with chronic fatigue syndrome
- Reduces epileptic seizures
- Helps protect against kidney disease and bladder infections. Dissolves kidney stones, and prevention of liver disease
- Supports thyroid function
- Applied topically forms a chemical barrier on the skin to ward of infection, reduces symptoms associated the psoriasis, eczema, and dermatitis
- Softens skin and helps relieve dryness and flaking
- Prevents wrinkles, sagging skin, and age spots; protection from ultraviolet radiation from the sun and helps control dandruff

Coconut oil, due to its unique absorption and metabolism characteristics, has been used therapeutically since the 1950s in the treatment of fat malabsorption, cystic fibrosis, epilepsy, weight control and to increase exercise performance. In a study done on triglyceride levels in healthy men, researchers found that:

"Medium chain triglycerides are readily hydrolyzed in the intestines and the fatty acids are transported directly to the liver via the portal venous system, in contrast to long-chain fatty acids (LCFAs), which are incorporated into chylomicrons for transport through the lymphatic system or peripheral circulation. Medium-chain fatty acids (MCFAs) do not require carnitine to cross the double mitochondrial membrane of the hepatocyte, thus they quickly enter the mitochondria and undergo rapid beta-oxidation, whereas most LCFAs are packaged into triglycerides in the hepatocyte. ... Mean triglyceride values after canola oil increased 47 percent above baseline while mean triglyceride values after MCT oil decreased 15 percent from baseline which is consistent with several other studies involving short- and longer-term feeding with MCT oil."[102, 103, 104]

This one dietary addition may prove far more beneficial to overall health than the use of cholesterol-lowering medications, while being free of their noxious side effects. However, moderation is the key here. I've had clients who developed gallbladder symptoms from the over-consumption of coconut oil. More is not better, especially for clients prone to gallbladder and pancreas issues or those who have had their gallbladder removed.

[102] (Nevin KG, 2004)
[103] (Calabrese C, 1999)
[104] (Cohen LA, 1998)

Cholesterol is essential for all animal life. It is primarily synthesized from simpler substances within the body. In a person weighing 150 pounds, typical total body cholesterol synthesis is about 1,000 mg per day and total body content is about 35 grams. Typical additional dietary intake in the United States is 200-300 mg per day. The body compensates for cholesterol intake by reducing the amount synthesized by the liver.

Cholesterol is excreted by the liver via the bile into the digestive tract; typically about half is reabsorbed by the small bowel back into the bloodstream. Cholesterol is necessary for building and maintain membranes; it regulates membrane fluidity over the range of physiological temperatures.

Within cell membranes, cholesterol functions in intracellular transport, cell signaling and nerve conduction. Cholesterol is a key component for the structure and function of endocytosis. Cholesterol is utilized in cell signaling processes, and in the formation of lipid rafts in the plasma membrane. In some neurons, a myelin sheath, rich in cholesterol, provides insulation for efficient conduction of impulses.

Cholesterol within cells is the precursor molecule in biochemical pathways. Cholesterol in the liver, converted to bile, is then stored in the gallbladder. Bile contains bile salts that solubilize fats in the digestive tract and aid in the absorption of intestinal fat molecules, as well as fat-soluble vitamins A, D, E and K. Cholesterol is an important forerunner molecule for the synthesis of Vitamin D and the steroid hormones, including adrenal hormones cortisol and aldosterone; the sex hormones progesterone, estrogens, and testosterone; and their derivatives. And current research suggests cholesterol acts as an antioxidant.

Cholesterol Controversy

In the 1950s, the lipid hypothesis (also known as the Diet-Heart hypothesis) was introduced by Dr. Ancel Keys. He proposed that saturated fat and high cholesterol play a role in the causation of atherosclerosis and cardiovascular disease. But do the studies actually support this? And are the studies worth the paper they are written on?

Dr. Keys was a brilliant researcher, but even the best scientists can become myopic. Data can be taken out of context or manipulated to fit the views of the researcher, reader or reporter. This is called cherry picking, and it happens every day. Many are guilty of it, whether they do it deliberately or not.

There are a great many reasons why I see the whole cholesterol boondoggle as a problem. Instead of citing all the technical issues with the Los Angelas VA study, Farmington and Oslo studies, however, I'll refer you to Ms. Minger, who has expertly crafted a book both informative, factual and entertaining. Denise Minger in her book *Death by Food Pyramid* does an excellent job of outlining the history, controversies, inconsistencies and politics of the great cholesterol saga. I highly recommend it to all interested in learning more about the topic.

The International Network of Cholesterol Skeptics responds to the Diet-Heart hypothesis with the following quote: "For decades, enormous human and financial resources have been wasted on the cholesterol campaign, more promising research areas have been neglected, producers and manufacturers of animal food all over the world have suffered economically, and millions of healthy people have been frightened and badgered into eating a tedious and flavorless diet or into taking potentially dangerous drugs for the rest of their lives. As the scientific evidence in support of the cholesterol campaign is non-existent, we consider it important to stop it as soon as possible."

Dr. Mary Enig, noted nutrition scientist, researcher and author, states the following in her book *Know Your Fats*: "Intake of cholesterol has no effect on cholesterol levels in 70% of people, and in the other third, it raises LDL and HDL similarly and does not affect the ratio. Intake of certain fatty acids increases cholesterol levels, but again this is more consistent with greater cholesterol synthesis. For example the most powerful increaser of total cholesterol is probably lauric acid, but lauric acid is also the most powerful reducer of the LDL-to-HDL-cholesterol ratio—this is consistent with lauric acid being burned for quick energy, thus increasing the energy state of the liver cell and allowing for greater cholesterol synthesis. In summary, eating traditional saturated and monounsaturated fats does not clog the liver and does not promote LDL oxidation."[105]

A study was released on August 14, 2012, claiming that eggs were as bad for arteries as cigarettes. This study was quickly disseminated over the vast media waves as "the gospel according to medicine and science." But Dr. Frank Hu, professor of nutrition and epidemiology at the Harvard School of Public Health, wrote, "[The study] did not measure or control other aspects of diet such as intakes of meats, fruits or vegetables and did not control for lifestyle factors such as physical

---

[105] (Duane Graveline, 2009)

inactivity. The data could be useful for generating some hypotheses, but it's hard to draw any causal conclusions."

He continues, "It's very worrisome that these authors of the egg-yolk-is-bad article have managed to come up with a fairly simple and relatively compelling story which will scare a lot of people away from eating egg yolks. The study has potentially grave consequences for people trying to improve their health and reduce their risk of stroke and heart disease—and that's because most people should be eating more eggs, and particularly the yolks, not fewer."

Dr. Stephanie Seneff and her research team at MIT are discovering compelling new findings concerning the role of dietary fat, cholesterol and our health. Her research is so counter to the current dietary dogma that it sounds shocking at first. She believes that Americans are actually suffering from a cholesterol deficiency rather than an excess. Seneff is concerned that studies like the above-mentioned only serve to confuse the public more about the role of dietary cholesterol. She believes that cholesterol has been wrongly vilified and that evidence actually supports that foods that contain high amounts of cholesterol—such as egg yolks and other animal proteins—are essential to improving heart health, maintaining a healthy weight and staving off many diet-related diseases.

An article about eggs on the Harvard School of Public Health's website reads, "While it's true that egg yolks have a lot of cholesterol—and so may weakly affect blood cholesterol levels—eggs also contain nutrients that may help lower the risk for heart disease, including protein, vitamins B12 and D, riboflavin and folate."

Dr. Frank Hu explains: "Much of the cholesterol in the blood is produced endogenously. However, dietary factors (fats and cholesterol) can influence serum cholesterol levels."

Many of the nutrients found in eggs are in the yolk. Egg yolk contains lecithin that helps the body digest fat and metabolize cholesterol; betaine and choline that lower homocysteine levels; glutathione, that fights cancer and prevents oxidation of LDL; lutein and zeaxanthin, which have been shown to reduce colon cancer; and biotin, a B vitamin necessary for healthy hair, skin and nerves.

Elevated cholesterol levels do not necessarily mean one is at greater risk for a heart attack, research shows. Greater than 60 percent of all heart attacks occur in people with normal cholesterol levels; the majority of persons with high cholesterol never suffer heart attacks.

Studies show high LDL (the so-called "bad cholesterol") and heart disease are not linked. In 2005, the *Journal of American Physicians and Surgeons* reported as many as half of the people who have heart disease have normal or desirable levels of LDL. In 2005, researchers found older men and women with high LDL live longer.

Leukemia and other forms of cancer are beneficially affected by lipids. Some of the research done on cholesterol uncovered an unintended consequence of increased omega-6 fats in the diet: increased cancer rates. Heart disease rates improved but not at the same speed for which study participants fell prey to cancer.[106] According to researchers at Penn State, a compound produced from fish oil that appears to target leukemia stem cells could lead to a cure for the disease.

"Research in the past on fatty acids has shown the health benefits of fatty acids on cardiovascular system and brain development, particularly in infants, but we have shown that some metabolites of Omega-3 have the ability to selectively kill the leukemia-causing stem cells in mice," said researchers. "The important thing is that the mice were completely cured of leukemia with no relapse."[107]

For my part, I will say that you should eat real foods, use moderation, don't smoke, limit your consumption of fake fats from fast food vendors and restaurants, get regular exercise of thirty minutes or more at one time, and find something to laugh about every day—even if it's at yourself.

If it comes in a commercial bag, box, can or jar it is likely to be more dangerous to your health than a Saturday morning meal of sunny-side-up eggs and real farm bacon.

---

[106] Universität Basel. "Lipids help to fight leukemia, study demonstrates." ScienceDaily. ScienceDaily, 16 June 2014. <www.sciencedaily.com/releases/2014/06/140616102437.htm>.
[107] Penn State. "Possible cure for leukemia found in fish oil." ScienceDaily. ScienceDaily, 23 December 2011. <www.sciencedaily.com/releases/2011/12/111222103112.htm>.

For years, we have been bombarded with talking points on how LDL cholesterol is not good for us. We have been told that it leads to heart disease and increases diabetes risk factors. At last, the media is reporting on what many of us have known all along: LDL cholesterol has a major role to play in the body.

"There is a link between low levels of so-called 'bad' low-density lipoprotein (LDL) cholesterol—that is, not enough of it—and increased cancer risk. Scientists at Tufts University found cancer patients who had never taken cholesterol-lowering drugs had lower LDL cholesterol levels for an average of about 19 years prior to their cancer diagnosis. It seems they were 'healthier'—according to the LDL demonizers—than those on statin medications.

"Previous studies looked at patients who did take cholesterol-lowering drugs; they also suggested a strong link between low LDL cholesterol levels and higher cancer risk." Said Scientists at Tufts University.

The "HDL cholesterol is good and LDL is bad" message of allopathic medicine is at the very least oversimplified. Cholesterol has many functions and LDL is needed to build new muscle, which is important as we age. LDL protects the brain, and low levels of it can escalate problems such as dementia and memory loss. As Dr. Joseph A. Mercola points out, "cholesterol is neither 'good' nor 'bad', and attempts to artificially lower cholesterol can be dangerous, in part because of severe side effects like muscle damage."

Everyone needs a villian, and for allopathic medicine in the 21st century, LDL cholesterol is listed as public enemy number one. The pharmacuetical industry benefits from a billion-dollar cholesterol drug market. "Statin drugs are taken by one in four Americans over the age of 45, and if sales drop Big Pharma would be in a serious financial crisis. In fact, as soon as the study's cancer findings were published, a heart 'expert' immediately warned 'statins used for LDL reduction should not be stopped if there is an appropriate use to lower heart disease risk.'"

Additionally, the standard of care that allopathic medical providers follow dictates that almost everyone utilize statins. In 2014, statin medications were being studied for their potential use in prostate cancer and diabetes therapies.[108, 109]

---

[108] Purdue University. "Cholesterol study suggests new diagnostic, treatment approach for prostate cancer." ScienceDaily. ScienceDaily, 4 March 2014. <www.sciencedaily.com/releases/2014/03/140304154633.htm>.

So allopathic medicine's advice is to continue the use of these "miracle drugs" even though they are linked to nerve damage, muscle damage, liver enzyme derangement, tendon problems, anemia, acidosis, cataracts, sexual dysfunction, depression, an increase in type 2 diabetes and now cancer.

In early 2014, information on statin drugs increasing the risk of type 2 diabetes by 48% in post-menopausal women was published online. Within hours, Medscape critics began efforts to erase the information from the public eye. Why is it so important for this news to be blocked?

As per usual, it has to do with money. Cholesterol-lowering statin drugs are one of the most frequently prescribed drugs on the market; in 2011, they were also approved for children. Information that hurts the bottom line has to be speedily buried and/or discredited. Thus, in the latter part of 2014, there were a flurry of publicized studies that loudly proclaimed, once again, that cholesterol medications are suitable for you.

Beginning in 2010, doctors were told to place all diabetics on statins to lower their risk of cardiovascular disease. Soon thereafter, Medscape presented information on the increased risk to female patients. The statistical information is from the Women's Health Initiative (WHI), the largest ongoing study of women's health in the United States. This study has thousands of participants.

"With this study, what we're seeing is that the risk of diabetes is particularly high in elderly women, and this risk is much larger than was observed in another previous meta-analysis," said senior investigator Dr. Yunsheng Ma (University of Massachusetts Medical School, Boston).

Annie Culver (Mayo Clinic, Rochester, MN), a pharmacist and lead investigator of the study, published online in the *Archives of Internal Medicine* that "close monitoring and an individualized risk-versus-benefit assessment is really a good thing, as well as an emphasis on continued lifestyle changes." She continued, "I think the risk [of diabetes] is definitely there for statins."

Dr. Ma, Culver and colleagues analyzed data from the WHI which included 153,840 postmenopausal women, aged 50-79. Information about statin use was obtained at enrollment and at year three; the current analysis includes data up until 2005. At baseline, 7.0% of women were taking statins, with 30% of women taking simvastatin, 27% taking lovastatin, 22% taking pravastatin, 12.5% taking

---

[109] Wake Forest Baptist Medical Center. "Cholesterol-lowering drugs may reduce cardiovascular death in type 2 diabetes." ScienceDaily. ScienceDaily, 16 July 2014.
<www.sciencedaily.com/releases/2014/07/140716123420.htm>.

fluvastatin and 8% taking atorvastatin. During the study period, 10,242 incident cases of diabetes were reported.

Dr. David Brownstein, MD, describes familial hypercholesterolemia (FH) as a genetic disorder characterized by high cholesterol levels—usually high LDL cholesterol levels. It affects less than 1% of the population. He has said that "the media and many prominent cardiologists would have you believe that having a diagnosis of familial hypercholesterolemia markedly increases the risk of cardiovascular disease and proves the hypothesis that elevated cholesterol levels are responsible for cardiovascular disease. However, the research actually disproves the hypothesis that elevated cholesterol levels are responsible for cardiovascular disease. Research has shown people with familial hypercholesterolemia live at least as long as people without the condition and fewer die from cancer and other diseases."

Lipitor®, an older statin drug, came off patent in 2009 when sales topped 13 billion dollars worldwide. Pfizer applied for a six-month extension of its patent after doing its studies of Lipitor® on younger patients. In the U.S. and EU, drug makers are allowed to apply for an additional six months of patent protection if they test their drug on children. Lipitor® was approved by the FDA for use in children and Pfizer® collected additional funds from its patent for an additional six months.

The side effects associated with statins include muscle pain, memory loss, brain dysfunction, premature aging, liver dysfunction, muscle breakdown and weakness, lowered immunity, fatigue, and blood sugar dysregulation and hormone dysfunction. More information about statin drugs can be found in *Drugs That Don't Work and Natural Therapies That Do (2nd Edition)* by Dr. David Brownstein, MD, and in *Lipitor the Memory Thief* by Duane Graveline.

In May of 2014, research from the University of Colorado caught my attention. At first it seemed very disconcerting, then it looked promising, and then just as quickly fell back to disconcerting. The published research goes as follows:

> *Results from a study by University of Colorado School of Medicine researchers show that pravastatin, a medicine widely used for treatment of high cholesterol, also slows down the growth of kidney cysts in children and young adults with autosomal dominant polycystic kidney disease (ADPKD).*
>
> *ADPKD is the most common potentially lethal hereditary kidney disease, affecting at least 1 in 1000 people. ADPKD is characterized by progressive kidney enlargement due to cyst growth, which results in loss of kidney function over time. At one time, ADPKD was termed 'adult' polycystic kidney disease but researchers are finding that clinical manifestations may be*

evident in childhood and even in utero. This strongly suggests that earlier intervention in childhood may have the greatest long-term effect on the progression of the disease.

"Based on our findings, we strongly recommend consideration of pravastatin use in ADPKD children and young adults unless there is a medical reason against taking a statin as determined by the patients' doctor,' says the co-principal investigator Melissa A. Cadnapaphornchai, MD, from CU School of Medicine's departments of pediatrics & medicine, who conducted the study with Robert W. Schrier, MD, at the CU School of Medicine. 'This is very exciting news as this is the first medication shown to help control kidney disease in ADPKD children."[110]

So why did this cause my alarm bells to go off? First, it was a small study of 110 children; their ages are not disclosed and the study does not follow the patients through puberty or monitor changes in their cognition or mental status (depression). There is no mention of dietary modifications or nutritional therapy to mitigate the kidney disease. I am left with a sinking feeling of what the future may look like for these children. From the pharmaceutical companies' perspective, it is good business. For every new condition a drug can be prescribed for, patents are extended and profits maximized. More patients on the medication for longer amounts of time equals more revenue for stockholders.

---

[110] University of Colorado Denver. "Statins given early decrease progression of kidney disease." ScienceDaily. ScienceDaily, 8 May 2014. <www.sciencedaily.com/releases/2014/05/140508133203.htm>.

Most Americans eat a diet that consists of little or no protein at breakfast, a bit of protein at lunch and an overabundance of protein at dinner. It is common, even for vegans and vegetarians, for one daily meal to be heavier in protein than others. Those who are chronically ill or elderly may only eat one meal a day and consume almost no protein at all.

As long as we get our recommended dietary allowance of about 60 grams it's all good, right? But are we really consuming 60 grams? Some are and others are not. The time of day we consume our protein is also problematic, according to research from a team of scientists at the University of Texas Medical Branch at Galveston, led by a muscle metabolism expert.

As it turns out, Dr. Barry Sears and others who promoted the "40-30-30" intake approach for blood sugar and weight control were right. Research from the University of Texas Medical Branch at Galveston reported in the spring of 2014 that:

> *This research shows the typical cereal or carbohydrate-dominated breakfast, a sandwich or salad at lunch and overly generous serving of meat/protein for dinner may not provide the best metabolic environment to promote healthy aging and maintenance of muscle size and strength.*

> *This study shows the potential for muscle growth is less than optimal when protein consumption is skewed toward the evening meal instead of being evenly distributed throughout the day.*

> *Age-related conditions such as osteoporosis (bone weakening) and sarcopenia (muscle wasting) do not develop all of a sudden. Rather they are insidious processes precipitated by suboptimal lifestyle practices, such as diet and exercise, in early middle age, the study states.*

> *The study's results were obtained by measuring muscle protein synthesis rates in healthy adults who consumed two similar diets that differed in protein distribution throughout the day. One of the diets contained 30 grams of protein at each meal, while the other contained 10 grams at breakfast, 15 grams at lunch and 65 grams at dinner. Lean beef was the primary nutrient-dense source of protein for each daily menu. Using blood samples and thigh muscle biopsies, the researchers then determined the subjects' muscle protein synthesis rates over a 24-hour period.*

The researchers provided volunteers with a generous daily dose of 90 grams of protein— consistent with the average amount currently consumed by healthy adults in the United States.

When study volunteers consumed the evenly distributed protein meals, their 24-hour muscle protein synthesis was 25 percent greater than subjects who ate according to the skewed protein distribution pattern. This result was not altered by several days of habituation to either protein distribution pattern.

The results of the study, Paddon-Jones points out, seem to show a more effective pattern of protein consumption is likely to differ dramatically from many Americans' daily eating habits.

"Usually, we eat very little protein at breakfast, a bit more at lunch and then consume a large amount at night. So we're not taking enough protein on board for efficient muscle building and repair during the day, and at night we're often taking in more than we can use. We run the risk of having this excess oxidized and ending up as glucose or fat."

A more efficient eating strategy for making muscle and controlling total caloric intake would be to shift some of the extra protein consumed at dinner to lunch and breakfast, Paddon-Jones points out. [111]

So how is it that red meat from cattle and other flesh foods have become such an integral, yet controversial part of the American diet?

"Although cattle have been domesticated for less than 10,000 years, they are the world's most valuable animal, as judged by their multiple contributions of draft power, meat, milk, hides and dung. Evidence for the domestication of cattle dates from between 8,000 and 7,000 years ago in southwestern Asia. Such dating suggests that cattle were not domesticated until cereal domestication had taken place, whereas sheep and goats entered the barnyard of humans with the beginning of agriculture. Domestication would have required a supply of animals that was initially met by capturing them from the wild. In the holding pens, some captive bulls and cows bred, and from these mating, calves were born. Their overall size was smaller, their temperament more docile; these aurochs born in captivity were kept as objects of sacrifice and allowed to breed. The next generation to follow reinforced the characteristics of the parents, and a gene pool that distinguished these bovines

[111] University of Texas Medical Branch at Galveston. "Full serving of protein at each meal helps one achieve maximum muscle health." ScienceDaily. ScienceDaily, 20 May 2014. <www.sciencedaily.com/releases/2014/05/140520133218.htm>.

from their wild forebears gradually formed. No longer were they aurochs, but rather cattle."[112]

As settlements and villages turned into cities, the livestock living in small pastures or pens contributed to poor air quality as the streets filled with animal and human excrement. By the Middle Ages, ordinances were passed to reduce the free-roaming animals and the wholesale slaughter of them. Just as the merchants of the day forced through edicts that suited them, they also knew how to ignore those that were not convenient. It would take butchers almost two hundred years to meet demands to sell meat by weight rather than by the piece. Hygiene in the Middle Ages was anything but stringent; the cook was at the mercies of her nose and the free use of spices to cover purification of meats.[113]

At the end of the Little Ice Age, the use of salt to preserve meat became more frequent. City-dwellers and seafarers could carry dried preserved meats instead of live animals. The quality and taste was less than the best.

The 1800s

From 1870 to 1890, livestock ranching was a thriving industry in the United States and Australia. Ranching provided the meat for boom towns, logging camps and railway development. Transportation of fresh foods, especially meat, was a problem; the dilemma of how to get fresh meat to European markets affected price and demand. Cattle were emaciated and week after 700 mile drives over dry lands and prairies. In the 1942 *Yearbook of Agriculture— Keeping Livestock Healthy*, sub-par livestock nutrition is cited as "responsible for significant economic losses" that lasted for decades.[114] The U.S. had been at the forefront of new meat canning processes, but much of the products were far from palatable. It wasn't long until the cattle were being rested in the grasslands to allow them time to fatten before harvest.

The Chinese used ice houses for the preservation of fresh food since the eighth century BC, but it was the Shaker ice houses and their expertise in layered insulation that made transportation in railroad ice cars possible over vast distances. In the 1850s a Glasgow man who had emigrated to Australia designed and improved an

---

[112] Cambridge World History of Food, Kenneth F. Kiple & Kriemhild Conee Ornelas [Cambridge University Press:Cambridge] 2000, Volume One (p. 490-1)
[113] Tannahill, R (1988) Food in History
[114] USDA Yearbook of Agriculture 1942 pg 645

ether-compressor which made ice manufacturing possible for the first time. This was the advent of refrigeration. [115]

Today

Markets and grocery stores offer a selection of fruits, vegetables and meat, flash frozen for our convenience. The consumer thinks very little about how the food got there, or where it came from. We assume that the quality of food at our fingertips is far superior to the food that was available to our ancestors; that it is cleaner, fresher and safer. However, every year food recalls result in millions of pounds of potentially dangerous foods being discarded.

In addition to the risks of contamination and spoilage, there is also the issue of added chemicals. According to a study from Sweden, men who eat moderate amounts of processed red meat may have an increased risk of incidence and death from heart failure, according to a study in *Circulation: Heart Failure*, a journal from the American Heart Association. Processed meats are preserved by smoking, curing, salting or adding preservatives. Examples include cold cuts (ham, salami), sausage, bacon and hot dogs.

"Processed red meat commonly contains sodium, nitrates, phosphates and other food additives, and smoked and grilled meats also contain polycyclic aromatic hydrocarbons, all of which may contribute to the increased heart failure risk," said Alicja Wolk, DMSc, senior author of the study and professor in the Division of Nutritional Epidemiology at the Institute of Environmental Medicine, Karolinska Institute in Stockholm, Sweden. "Unprocessed meat is free from food additives and usually has a lower amount of sodium."[116]

Over a century ago, the federal government passed the Meat Inspection Act of 1906 to protect consumers from tainted meat products. Back then, meat was commonly adulterated with substances such as sulfate, boric acid, formaldehyde, coal tar and saltpeter.

It wasn't just the meat—questionable additives like coal dust and kerosene were used to fool consumers into thinking that green coffee beans were roasted (if it was

---

[115] (Tannahill, 1988)
[116] Joanna Kaluza, Agneta Åkesson, and Alicja Wolk. Processed and Unprocessed Red Meat Consumption and Risk of Heart Failure: A Prospective Study of Men. Circ Heart Fail., June 12 2014 DOI: 10.1161/CIRCHEARTFAILURE.113.000921

even coffee at all!). It wasn't until 1965 that manufacturers were required to list ingredients on products meant for human consumption.[117]

In 2010, the great "pink slime" scandal erupted. The Modesto Meat Company recalled about one million pounds of ground beef products after seven people were sickened by *E. coli* contamination. The U.S. Department of Agriculture announced that the Valley Meat Company had sold the potentially contaminated meat in California, Texas, Oregon, Arizona and internationally.[118, 119]

Suddenly, news about "pink slime" was everywhere. On *FoodNavigator.com*, a website for those in the food industry, I saw the headline: "Pink slime: Safe, nutritious and icky." It went on to say that "scary junk science about ammonium hydroxide has led to a safe, nutritious product being pulled from stores. Beef Products Inc, the nation's leading manufacturer of 'pink slime' aka lean finely textured beef—is suspending production of the product at three of four plants after major retailers said they would stop buying it. The move follows a storm of media hysteria spewed forth onto a largely ignorant public."

The news report went on to say that "if the Beef Products manufacturing company can't clear itself from this pink slime PR mess, it will mean 1.5 million cattle will need to be slaughtered to meet demands for ground beef, pink slime free."

What about the ammonium hydroxide? The Material Safety Data Sheet reports: "Very hazardous in case of skin contact (corrosive, irritant, permeator), of eye contact (irritant), of ingestion. Non-corrosive to the eyes. Non-corrosive for lungs. Liquid or spray mist may produce tissue damage particularly on mucous membranes of eyes, mouth and respiratory tract. Skin contact may produce burns. Inhalation of the spray mist may produce severe irritation of respiratory tract, characterized by coughing, choking, or shortness of breath. Severe over-exposure can result in death.

"Inflammation of the eye is characterized by redness, watering and itching. Skin inflammation is characterized by itching, scaling, reddening, or, occasionally, blistering. Repeated or prolonged exposure to the substance can produce target organs damage. Ingestion: If swallowed, do not induce vomiting unless directed to do so by medical personnel. Never give anything by mouth to an unconscious person. Loosen tight clothing such as a collar, tie, belt or waistband. Get medical attention immediately."

---

[117] What's Cooking Uncle Sam, National Archives page 42
[118] (Tribune, 2010)
[119] (News)

I am thankful for the availability of real meat through local ranchers. I've never once had my T-bones recalled due to contamination.

So What About Fish?

Do you buy fish from the store? How about that favorite basket of fish 'n' chips from the local fast food joint? Are you sure that it's the fish the menu or label says it is?

A report from the ocean conservation group Oceana reveals that there is a decent chance the fish you just bought is not what you think it is. Between 2010 and 2012, Oceana took 1,215 seafood samples from 674 retail outlets in 21 states. When they tested the DNA, they found that 33 percent were mislabeled. Sushi vendors and grocery stores were the most likely outlets to sell mislabeled food, though Oceana says the fraud can happen before it reaches them.

Seafood mislabeling is common in cities like New York and Boston, where people eat a lot of fish. The report, released on February 21, 2013, shows fraudulent labeling is happening across the country, and is just as likely to occur in Texas and Colorado as in Boston or New York. Some 49 percent of the retail outlets sampled in Austin and Houston sold mislabeled seafood; in Colorado, 36 percent did. The highest mislabeling rates occurred with snapper and tuna: 87 and 59 percent. Only seven of the 120 samples of red snapper purchased nationwide were actually red snapper, the report found.

So what's the big deal? For one, it's a form of swindling to sell a cheap fish like tilapia for a red snapper price. Additionally, the practice can put consumers at risk when species such as king mackerel, which is high in mercury, or escolar, which contains a naturally occurring toxin that can cause gastrointestinal problems, are marketed as grouper and white tuna, respectively.

The U.S. now imports 90 percent of its seafood; less than 2 percent is inspected for fraud. That means would-be fraudsters have a lot of opportunities to make substitutions.

The Food and Drug Administration regularly updates its list of seafood approved for sale. In 2012 alone, 19 new species were added to the list, including cornetfish, sampa and claresse. Ever heard of these?

So dust off your poles and fishing gear or take a drive to the coast and visit a U.S.-owned fish cannery. Buy fresh fish off the boat and can or freeze it yourself and support our local U.S. fisheries.

Be especially wary of fish from Thailand, Vietnam and China. These countries have posted health advisories to their own citizens regarding the dangers of eating their domestically farmed fish.

Protein Drinks

Protein drinks should not be used as food replacements. Real food contains a symphony of nutrients that the human body needs to keep blood sugars, the immune system, muscle tissue and brain function in optimum shape. Protein powders are used in clinical settings to prevent muscle wasting in cancer patients and the elderly or to help patients regain control of unhealthy blood sugars and reduce obesity. In the sports arena, protein products are used to bulk up. They promise "hope in a can" that you too can look like this stud muffin on the label or in the body builder ad.

The convenience aspect of these products is alluring to those of us trying to keep our weight under control while working long hours. But looks can be deceiving and there is very little truth in advertising.

Here is some of the information found in a *Consumer Reports* article:

"Out of 15 top protein drink products sent to an independent assay lab, all were found to contain some form of heavy metals; most prominent were arsenic, mercury, lead and cadmium. Some of the products contained what were considered low to moderate levels, others like EAS, and Muscle Milk were found to contain high levels of two or more of the heavy metals.

These heavy metals damage the liver, endocrine glands and the kidneys; these are also the organs that process protein.

The report goes on to say the age group most actively using these commercial products are teens from the age of 12 to 18 and they will use as much as 4-8 times the label serving size, ensuring that even protein products listed in the low toxicity level become dangerous. EAS® Myoplex Original Rich Chocolate Shake contained 16.9 mcg of arsenic and 5.1mcg of cadmium. Cadmium is of particular concern because of how it displaces iodine from cell receptor sites and accumulates in the kidneys taking over 20 years for the body to eliminate." [120]

---

[120] (Report, July 2010)

When we look at the research and current dietary recommendations, we may conclude that we are poisoning ourselves with protein. But let's look a little deeper into history and human physiology.

Man has a long tradition of eating meat (but not protein powders). There are still, to this day, populations that live almost entirely on meat and animal by-products like fat, milk, blood and cheese. These are real foods that contain a host of vitamins, minerals and amino acids that our DNA structures know what to do with. Protein extracted from vegetable sources like soy, wheat (gluten), rice and corn are not complete proteins and are very difficult for the human digestive system to break down.

Asian societies learned long ago that in order for soy protein to be useful it had to be fermented or predigested and even then, other foods were necessary to prevent side effects to the thyroid, prostate and breasts. The average Japanese consumes over 15 mg of iodine through seafood and sea vegetables daily. The iodine protects against the excess estrogens and goitrogen properties of the soy. In addition to soy, Asians consume meat, bones, eyes, glands, skin and internal organs, which provides them with a broad range of amino acids and nutrients. By the way, the Japanese refuse to eat American soy foods and do not let Monsanto sell GMO soy in their country. I wonder why?

Most Americans eat too much and eat too many manufactured foods. Overloading with any one food can lead to health problems, especially for those who are still developing. If you are using a protein product, research the ingredients and the brand you selected; or, buy from a practitioner who has investigated the product. Use them as a short-term or fill-in supplement, not as a meal replacement.

Teach your teens how to cook real food and how to buy good meat and fresh foods. Home economics class is not going to do it for you (it hasn't been taught in schools since the 1980s). Make family meals or cook for a family event that everyone can get involved in at least once a week. As a parent, don't let your son use protein powders without supervision; they're going to need their kidneys and liver for many years yet.

Ketogenic diets—diets high in protein—may not be for everyone. However, a study reported in December 2014 by the American Epilepsy Society illustrates that the ketogenic approach is highly beneficial for clients with epilepsy.

Researchers at John Hopkins University conducted a four-year study at their Adult Epilepsy Diet Center. From August 2010 to August 2014, the authors followed 134 adults with epilepsy, including 21 participants who were already following a ketogenic diet (KD). Of the 113 adults new to diet therapy, 100 qualified as having drug-resistant epilepsy (tried 2 or more anti-seizure drugs with continued seizures). Seventy-eight began a modified Atkins diet (MAD), 2 began an enteral version of the KD in addition to MAD by mouth as tolerated, and 20 chose not to begin diet therapy or have yet to start. A neurologist and dietitian provided the initial evaluation, education and follow-up for all participants.

Their findings suggest that dietary therapy may be beneficial to some adults with epilepsy. Of the 78 patients with drug-resistant epilepsy who began a MAD, the median seizure frequency was 10 seizures per week. The authors analyzed one month of data from 78 study participants and found that 43 (55%) had a greater than 50% seizure reduction. Of these, 28 (36%) patients became seizure-free. Patients who became seizure-free had been diagnosed with focal epilepsy (17), generalized epilepsy (10, including 5 with juvenile myoclonic epilepsy), and Doose syndrome (1). In addition, fifty-eight participants supplied three-month calendars of self-reported seizure activity. Of these fifty-eight patients, 28 had a seizure reduction greater than 50% and 14 became seizure-free.[121, 122, 123, 124]

To determine how much protein you personally need requires a little math

A female with low to moderate activity level, weighing 135 pounds, requires between 86 and 143 grams of protein daily for normal blood sugar and metabolic function. If she is very active, her protein requirements increase.

1.5 grams (gr) of protein are required to make 1 pound of muscle.

The formula: Divide body weight by .4536, then divide that answer by 2. This number will equal the number of grams per day of protein needed for health.

(135 /.4536 = 297 / 2 = 149 g / 3 (number of average meals daily) = 49 g approximate total protein per meal = approx. 3 oz (1 oz = 28.34 g)

[121] American Epilepsy Society (AES). "Adults and epilepsy diets: A novel therapy." ScienceDaily. ScienceDaily, 8 December 2014. <www.sciencedaily.com/releases/2014/12/141208144152.htm>.
[122] American Academy of Neurology (AAN). "Low carb, high fat diets may reduce seizures in tough-to-treat epilepsy." ScienceDaily. ScienceDaily, 29 October 2014. <www.sciencedaily.com/releases/2014/10/141029203747.htm>.
[123] Johns Hopkins Medicine. "Fasting may benefit patients with epilepsy." ScienceDaily. ScienceDaily, 6 December 2012. <www.sciencedaily.com/releases/2012/12/121206203122.htm>.
[124] Michael V. Accardi, Bryan A. Daniels, Patricia M.G.E. Brown, Jean-Marc Fritschy, Shiva K. Tyagarajan, Derek Bowie. Mitochondrial reactive oxygen species regulate the strength of inhibitory GABA-mediated synaptic transmission. Nature Communications, 2014; 5 DOI: 10.1038/ncomms4168

Edible eggs

Eggs are one of those foods Americans have been eating for a long time: eggs benedict, deviled eggs, egg salad, boiled, fried, scrambled and poached eggs. Yet the health benefits of eggs have been questioned.

In 2013, NPR reported on how the color of eggs in the United States compares to eggs from other countries. While the story did little to encourage individuals to eat farm-pastured eggs, it did remind me of my 4-H days and conversations over poultry feed and commercial egg production.

Eggs get their color from the feed given to the birds. Corn and wheat add a more yellow coloring to the yolks. But chickens are far from vegetarian. I have always found it interesting that poultry is allowed in strict Jewish diets—after all, chickens break most of the dietary guidelines for food animals, as do ducks and geese.

Chickens prefer a good juicy bug to grain, and they love baby grass. It is these foods that add nutritional value to eggs. Yes, they'll gobble up grains and seeds, but what they really want is found in a three-day-old cow pie or compost pile. Just like cows, their digestive system was not designed to subsist solely on grain.

Everything an animal eats becomes part of their flesh and DNA. If you are allergic to wheat, corn or soy and consume animals that were fed on these grains, you could suffer an allergic or inflammatory response that could possibly lead to chronic illness.

Here is an example: I have a 57-year-old client who has violent reactions to corn and dairy. Most commercial milk comes from cows that were fed corn. Also, when this client eats store-bought eggs, regardless of whether they are cage-free, organic or commercial, he immediately suffers from gas, cramping and diarrhea. When this client eats truly free-range eggs from the chickens fed only cracked peas and whatever they can find on their own, there is no distress. Are you seeing the connection here?

It isn't just about what we eat, but also about what is consumed by what we eat. The same applies to our soils and vegetables, fruits and fish.

Next, we run into the fairytale world of medical myth. For years, doctors told patients to stop eating eggs because they are high in cholesterol and could lead to heart disease.

On July 19, 2013, a study was published that would make my great-grandmother smack her forehead. To her, it was common sense that eggs were good for a growing child. The news headline read: "Eating Eggs Is Not Linked to High Cholesterol in Adolescents, Study Suggests."

It went on to state that "Although in the late 20th century it was maintained that eating more than two eggs a week could increase cholesterol, in recent years experts have begun to refute this myth. Now, a new study has found that eating more eggs is not associated with higher serum cholesterol in adolescents, regardless of how much physical activity they do."

There is more. Let's look at the information from Dr. Niva Shapira of Tel Aviv University's School of Health Professions. In a study published August 2, 2011, she discovers that eggs are not created equal. "Eggs high in omega-6 fatty acids heighten cholesterol's tendency to oxidize, which forms dangerous plaque in arteries. Dr. Shapira's research shows eggs laid by hens with healthier feed can lessen oxidation of LDL (low-density lipoprotein), the body's 'bad cholesterol'.

"'But healthier eggs cost more,' Dr. Shapira says. 'The price of chicken feed varies from region to region, and in many areas, feed containing products high in omega-6 fatty acids, such as wheat, corn or maize, soy and their oils, are much cheaper for egg producers to purchase.'"

Americans, Japanese, Australians and Scandinavians tend to wash and refrigerate their eggs. Soon after a chicken lays an egg, American producers put them straight into a machine that shampoos them with soap and hot water. The steamy shower leaves the shells squeaky clean. But it also compromises them, by washing away a barely visible sheen that naturally envelops each egg.

"The egg is a marvel in terms of protecting itself, and one of the protections is this coating, which prevents them from being porous," says food writer Michael Ruhlman, author of *Egg: A Culinary Exploration of the World's Most Versatile Ingredient.*[125] After sharing this information with a friend newly transplanted to the Czech Republic, they replied back that they would quit complaining about the bits of feathers and bird poop on their eggs.

So the bottom line is to buy from the farmers' market or directly from a local farmer. Look them in the eye and ask if they are feeding commercial egg maker or do their birds free range? Are they washing the eggs or wiping them off? I know my egg providers by name and sight. They live in our community and I know they depend

[125] http://www.npr.org/blogs/thesalt/2014/09/11/336330502/why-the-u-s-chills-its-eggs-and-most-of-the-world-doesnt

financially on the quality of the food they produce, just like I depend on it for my health.

Talkin' Turkey

Today's domesticated turkey is descended from the wild turkey. It was the Mesoamericans who first domesticated the wild turkey. For the Aztecs it was an important source of protein; the feathers were used for decorative purposes. Additional evidence suggests the Hopi Indians may have domesticated the turkey even before the Aztecs.

Spanish explorers, who had found them among the Aztecs and other Mesoamerican peoples, introduced the turkey to Europe. After being introduced to Europe, many distinct turkey breeds were developed. In the early 20th century, advances were made in the breeding of turkeys, resulting in varieties such as the Beltsville Small White.

Turkeys are traditionally eaten as the main course in Christmas feasts (stuffed turkey), as well as for Thanksgiving in the United States and Canada. This tradition has its origins in modern times, rather than colonial. Before the 20th century, pork ribs were the most common food on the holiday menu, as the animals were usually slaughtered in November. Turkeys were once so abundant in the wild that they were eaten throughout the year. The food was considered commonplace, whereas pork ribs were rarely available outside of the Thanksgiving-New Year season. Turkey has also displaced, to a certain extent, the traditional Christmas roast goose or beef of the United Kingdom and Europe.

Before World War II, turkey was a luxury in the United Kingdom. Goose or beef was featured in the typical Christmas dinner. In Charles Dickens' *A Christmas Carol*, Bob Cratchit had a goose before Scrooge bought him a turkey. Intensive turkey farming from the late 1940s dramatically reduced the price, shifting turkey to the most common Thanksgiving and Christmas dinner meat. With the availability of refrigeration, whole turkeys could be shipped frozen to distant markets. Disease control increased production, allowing turkey to be eaten year-round.

Turkeys are sold sliced and ground, as well as "whole" in a manner similar to chicken, with the head, feet and feathers removed. Sliced turkey is frequently used as a sandwich meat or served as cold cuts. Ground turkey is frequently marketed as a beef substitute.

Wild turkeys, while technically the same species as domesticated turkeys, have a very different taste from farm-raised turkeys. Almost all of the meat is dark, even the breast, and it has a more intense flavor. The flavor can also vary seasonally with changes in forage, often leaving wild turkey meat with a gamier flavor in late summer due to the greater number of insects in its diet. Wild turkey that has fed predominantly on grass and grain has a milder flavor. Older heritage breeds also differ in flavor.

Some states in the south have a thriving poultry industry. Arkansas is one such state. As you drive along mountain roads that take you from ridge top to holler, you see on the wide-open ridge tops large, half-dome barns with huge fans at each end and shutters that open on the sides. These neat and tidy farms are marked with signs on the gate or fence post that read Tyson or Butter Ball. The agricultural income is essential to the rural areas of Arkansas. The mega-farming model is not the ideal, but neither is starvation and poverty.

Approximately two to four billion pounds of poultry feathers are produced every year by the poultry industry. Most are ground into a protein source for ruminant animal feed. Researchers at the United States Department of Agriculture (USDA) have patented a method of removing the stiff quill from the fibers making up the feather. As this is a potential supply of natural fibers, the Philadelphia University School of Engineering and Textiles has researched ways to blend turkey fibers with nylon to form a yarn for knitting, textiles and clothing.

Health Benefits

Turkey contains a host of amino acids, with particularly high levels of L-lysine and leucine. Wild turkey also contains essential fatty acids, iron, chromium and zinc with the peptide anserine. The greatest levels of essential fatty acids are found in the skin at 39.3%. Roasted turkey contains about 29% protein per 100 grams of meat that is almost 40% less than an equal amount of soy protein. This may partially account for the dangers of soy isolate products and their potential to cause kidney and liver damage.

Noted researchers like Russell L. Blaylock, MD, believe that many of the chemicals that are added to food could damage a critical part of the brain that controls hormones, which could lead to endocrine problems. They are called excitotoxins and include artificial colors (FD&C colors), sodium nitrite and nitrate, BHT (butylated hydroxytohicne), saccharin, MSG (monosodium glutamate), aspartame, caffeine, propylene glycol, sulfites (especially sodium bisulfite), sulfur dioxide, BVO (Brominated Vegetable Oil) and BPA (bisphenol A, invented in the 1960s). [126, 127, 128]

We may be religiously working out, taking supplements and eating right, but feel as though we are losing our edge. This may be due to neurotoxins hidden in our foods, including those labeled organic and natural. These ingredients often cause serious reactions, including migraines, insomnia, asthma, depression, anxiety, aggression, chronic fatigue and even ALS. They may be responsible for the growing numbers of children diagnosed with ADHD and autism.

Evidence strongly suggests that artificial sweeteners in diet soft drinks, gums, candy and foods may cause brain tumors to develop. The number of brain tumors reported since the widespread introduction of artificial sweeteners has risen dramatically. In addition, obesity has skyrocketed.

Monosodium glutamate (MSG) is probably the best known of the neurotoxins; it is sometimes disguised as yeast extract, maltodextrin, carrageenan, hydrolyzed vegetable protein, dough conditioners, seasonings and spices. Hazardous chemicals are added to virtually all restaurant food, from McDonald's® to the most exclusive gourmet dining spots. While 1 out of every 4 people is sensitive to neurotoxic food additives, only 1 in 250 is aware that these additives are the source of the reactions they are having.

MSG is natural and has been used in Asian cooking for decades as a flavor enhancer. During World War II, American food manufacturers began using MSG to improve the taste of C-rations (C stands for "combat") for the troops. Originally isolated from seaweed, MSG is now made by fermenting corn, potatoes and rice. MSG is naturally present in high levels in tomatoes and Parmesan cheese. These natural foods have

---

[126] (Deanna M. Minich, 2009)
[127] (Ruth Winter, 1999)
[128] http://www.mayoclinic.org/healthy-living/nutrition-and-healthy-eating/expert-answers/bpa/faq-20058331

built-in protection in the form of antioxidants to offset the damage from naturally occurring MSG. But man-made or modern MSG is highly dangerous to health. An early study reported the inner layer of the retina was destroyed in neonatal rats receiving a single exposure to MSG. This is an amazing finding considering that humans are more than 5 times more sensitive to MSG than rats.

The definition of "natural flavor" under the Code of Federal Regulations is "the essential oil, oleoresin, essence or extractive, protein hydrolysate, distillate, or any product of roasting, heating or enzymolysis, which contains the flavoring constituents derived from a spice, fruit or fruit juice, vegetable or vegetable juice, edible yeast, herb, bark, bud, root, leaf or similar plant material, meat, seafood, poultry, eggs, dairy products, or fermentation products thereof, whose significant function in food is flavoring rather than nutritional" (21CFR101.22).

So what about the flavorings used in organic foods? Foods certified by the National Organic Program (NOP) must be grown and processed using organic farming methods without synthetic pesticides, bioengineered genes, petroleum-based fertilizers and sewage sludge-based fertilizers. Organic livestock cannot be fed antibiotics or growth hormones.

The term "organic" is not synonymous with "natural." The USDA's Food Safety and Inspection Service (FSIS) defines "natural" as "a product containing no artificial ingredient or added color and is only minimally processed may be labeled natural." Most foods labeled natural, including its flavorings, are not subject to government controls beyond the regulations and health codes.[129, 130, 131]

Food and beverage companies use food additives because they make you crave more of what tastes so good. They cause nerve cells to cry out for repeated stimulation, and keep you buying and consuming more of their products. If you want to avoid neurotoxic additives, know there is more to it than looking for MSG or artificial sweetener on the label. Even if products call themselves "all-natural" or "organic", it may still contain neurotoxic additives. There is no way to know unless you are willing to take the time to read the label closely, and even call the manufacturer to clarify the label information.

Excitotoxins have been found to dramatically promote cancer growth and metastasis. In fact, one excitotoxin researcher noticed that, when cancer cells were exposed to glutamate, they became more mobile. MSG also causes a cancer cell to become more mobile, which in turn enhances metastasis, or spread.[132]

According to Dr. Blaylock, a dramatic and statistically significant increase in the related cancers of lymphoma and leukemia, along with several histological types of lymphomas (especially of primary lymphoma of the brain) are associated with MSG and aspartame.They act as either a co-carcinogen or a primary carcinogen. Dr. Blaylock believes the culprit is the formaldehyde breakdown product.

A study conducted in Spain showed that radiolabeled aspartame broke down into formaldehyde; it was then seen binding to DNA, where it produced both single and double-strand DNA breakage.

Researchers discovered that outside of the brain, "there are numerous glutamate receptors in all organs and tissues. The entire GI tract, from the esophagus to the colon, has numerous glutamate receptors. The entire electrical conducting system of a heart is replete with multiple types of glutamate receptors. The lungs, the ovaries, all the reproductive systems and sperm itself, adrenal glands, bones and even the pancreas are all controlled by glutamate receptors. They act and operate exactly like the glutamate receptors in the brain."

When you are consuming MSG, the level of glutamate in the blood can rise as high as 20-fold, resulting in very high glutamate levels in the blood after eating a meal containing MSG. You're stimulating all of the glutamate receptors. Some people get explosive diarrhea and dyspepsia, because it stimulates the receptors in the esophagus and small bowel. Others may develop irritable bowel, or worsen pre-existing irritable bowel. In the case of GERD reflux, MSG and aspartame increase symptomology resulting in increased episodes and severity. The cardiac system is also affected by these potent chemicals; glutamate receptors being activated may explain the rise in sudden cardiac death."[133]

Low magnesium levels are found in all of these cases. When magnesium levels are low, the glutamate receptors become hypersensitive. Athletes in particular, if not supplementing with magnesium, are prone to sudden cardiac death.

Many brands of infant and toddler foods contain caseinate hydrolyzed protein, soy extracts and broth, which are all a significant source of glutamate.

---

[132] (Russell Blaylock, 2009)
[133] (Russell Blaylock, 2009)

Soy extracts are by far the worst, not only because of the GMO issue but because soybeans naturally have one of the highest glutamate levels of any plant products. When hydrolyzed, as in soy protein isolates, glutamate is released. The glutamate levels are higher than many other MSG-containing products. A 25-year study on vegetarians who consumed a high amount of soy products involved serial CT scans of their brains. The people who consumed the most soybean products had the greatest incidence of dementia and brain atrophy.

Researchers have shown that there are glutamate receptors on both sides of the blood-brain barrier and that when you expose these receptors to glutamate, it opens up the barrier. As you get older, your barrier becomes less impermeable. Almost all Alzheimer's patients have incompetent barriers. Heat stroke, seizures, autoimmune disorders and multiple sclerosis are all associated with an inefficient blood-brain barrier.[134, 135]

Brominated Vegetable Oil (BVO)

One of the great things about the Internet is it allows me to keep track of European food and manufacturing standards. Since they are more intolerant of GMO foods and other Monsanto products, I get to read studies that never make it into U.S. news. One example is when a German professor told BeverageDaily.com that "the best solution to eliminate concerns regarding brominated vegetable oil (BVO) from U.S. soft drinks is a voluntary ban." The FDA response to this is "changing the interim approval status of BVO would require the expenditure of the FDA's limited resources and is not a public health priority for the agency."

BVO displaces iodine, a necessary mineral for thyroid function and for the prevention of breast and prostate cancers. Excess bromine may cause fatigue, irritability, memory loss, sleep disorders and weakness. Continued excessive consumption of bromine may cause acne, confusion, depression, drowsiness, delirium, hallucinations, irritability, psychosis, schizophrenia and stupor.

BVO is found in Mountain Dew®, Fanta Orange® and many processed foods; it is also used as a flame retardant in plastics and is banned for use in food in Europe and Japan. Maybe we should listen to the German researcher instead of the FDA?

---

[134] (Russell L. Blaylock, Sweet Deception, 2006)
[135] (Russell L. Blaylock, Excitotoxins - the taste that kills, 1997)

Throughout 2011 and 2012, every time a study came out linking sugar or chemicals with brain disorders like ADHD and depression, the media jumped on the food industry's bandwagon about "junk science".

A 2012 study linked fast food consumption with a greater risk of depression. This study has been published in the *Public Health Nutrition Journal* and was headed by scientists from the University of Las Palmas de Gran Canaria and the University of Granada. An excerpt reads: "eating commercial baked goods (fairy cakes, croissants, doughnuts, etc.) and fast food (hamburgers, hotdogs and pizza) is linked to depression; the results reveal consumers of fast food, compared to those who eat little or none, are 51% more likely to develop depression. Furthermore, a dose-response relationship was observed. In other words this means that the more fast food you consume, the greater the risk of depression.".

Detoxification

As many as 80,000 commercial and industrial chemicals are now used in the United States; hundreds more are introduced into the marketplace on a weekly basis. Many of these chemicals are used in food packaging and commercial foods as flavor enhancers and preservatives. The majority of these chemicals were never in our diet prior to 1980. The lack of information available on the effects of these substances on human health at chronic low-dose exposure is concerning. Food manufacturing companies are not required to provide long-term research on the effects of these chemicals. Furthermore, the effect of exposure from multiple substances simultaneously, which is the norm, is virtually unknown.

A recent study by the Agency for Toxic Substances and Disease Registry (ATSDR) found that "when examining the components of 15 combinations and how they may interact, they predicted that 41% of them would have additive effects, 20% would have synergistic effects, but for 24% they did not have the minimum information necessary to predict the effects. ... It has been estimated that at current funding levels, it would take 1,000 years to adequately document the health effects of the chemicals commonly encountered in commerce and industry." (*Tracking chemical exposures and human health. Environ Health Perspect. 2003;111(7):A374-375*).

Considering the effect of one chemical at a time is no longer sufficient to understanding the biochemical pathways affected and the health risk outcome. The Centers for Disease Control (CDC) published data on the levels of selected persistent organic pollutants (POPs), "a category of toxins which includes dioxins, phthalates, PDBEs, PCBs, etc.—and found that among a representative sample of the U.S.

population, some toxins were present in essentially every individual over the age of 12. ... An analysis of NHANES data found up to a 38-fold adjusted increase in risk for diabetes prevalence in those with the highest levels," and increased risk has been documented additionally for cardiovascular disease, insulin resistance, impaired neurological development, learning and attention deficit disorders, endometriosis, and deficits in the hypothalamic pituitary-thyroid axis. In a nutshell, all of these chemicals we are exposed to daily are making us sick.

Damage is caused by a variety of mechanisms. Most toxins increase oxidative stress by poisoning enzymes, directly damaging DNA or cellular membranes and acting as endocrine disruptors. For example, the toxic metal cadmium increases oxidative damage by causing the formation of free radicals and by directly poisoning several enzymes which reduce oxidative stress, including catalase, glutathione reductase, and the most abundant cellular antioxidant, glutathione.

Unfortunately, no protocol exists for the testing of most toxins. Most detoxification programs focus exclusively on the liver, but the role of the GI tract is crucial because the greatest portion of the toxic load on the liver comes from the bowel.

To effectively eliminate toxins, the body goes through a series of processes that must occur in sequence. While detoxifying, it is important to support the body with adequate levels of vital vitamins, minerals, amino acids, phytochemicals and dietary fiber.

A number of nutrients have been shown to repair damaged intestinal lining and regulate the elimination of toxins:

- ✓ L-glutamine: primary amino acid source for intestinal cells, glutamine has been shown to regulate intercellular junction integrity.
- ✓ Probiotics: the greatest factor in determining intestinal integrity is the health of the microbial flora.
- ✓ N-acetyl glucosamine (NAG): provides a substrate for the repair of gut tissues.
- ✓ Zinc: deficiency has been shown to disrupt cells formation, alter membrane permeability, impair immune function and cause intestinal ulceration.
- ✓ Antioxidants (vitamin C, vitamin E, beta-carotene, grape seed extract and milk thistle extract): protect the GI tract from oxidant damage, and help with hepatic detoxification of compounds associated with intestinal dysfunction.
- ✓ Quercetin: critical to intestinal integrity, acts through a number of mechanisms.

- ✓ Highly digestible protein and low-allergy water soluble fiber: known to restore intestinal health and aid in the elimination of chemicals.
- ✓ N-acetyl cysteine: increase the urinary excretion of several toxic metals in proportion to body burden, especially mercury. It has been shown to increase hepatic glutathione, assisting in the detoxification of acetaminophen.
- ✓ Chlorella: proven to reduce the absorption of specific toxins in the GI tract, such as dioxins, as well as the reabsorption of stored dioxins. Supplementation with chlorella has been shown to reduce the maternal transfer of dioxins in breast milk.
- ✓ Milk thistle: a powerful hepatoprotective agent, and a potent antioxidant against environmental toxins.
- ✓ Broccoli : supports several phase 2 metabolic pathways, has been shown to reduce harmful estrogens, leading to reduced breast, prostate and cervical cancer risk.
- ✓ Lipoic acid: lipoic acid is a heavy metal chelator, and restores glutathione levels.
- ✓ Green tea: shown to protect the liver from alcohol.

Airborne Allergies

Approximately 38% of the population of Western nations experience allergies. Mild allergies like hay fever are highly prevalent in the human population and cause symptoms such as allergic conjunctivitis, itchiness and runny nose. Hay fever involves inflammation of the nose that occurs as a result of an allergic reaction to wind-borne pollens, grasses or weeds. Hay fever is caused primarily by antigens that initiate an allergic response. Some of the many antigens that can initiate hay fever include: house dust, animal hair, dust mites, fungus spores, feathers, powders, pesticides, and tree and grass pollen.

"An allergy is a disorder of the immune system often referred to as *atopy*. Allergic reactions occur to normally harmless environmental substances known as allergens; these reactions are acquired, predictable and rapid. Strictly, allergy is one of the four forms of hypersensitivity and is called *type I* (or *immediate*) hypersensitivity. It is characterized by excessive activation of certain white blood cells called *mast cells* and *basophils* by a type of antibody known as IgE, resulting in an extreme inflammatory response. Common allergic reactions include eczema, hives, hay fever, asthma, food allergies, and reactions to the venom of stinging insects such as wasps and bees."

What To Do?

Not everyone can take over-the-counter antihistamines due to high blood pressure, drug interactions or sensitivities to the chemicals they contain. If you are one of these individuals or you choose to avoid drug use for other reasons here are some suggestions for reducing hay fever naturally:

- ❖ **Bee Pollen**: Bee pollen has been used for centuries in China for seasonal allergies. It dries up the nasal cavity and slows or stops that annoying post nasal drip that leads to nagging coughing, sore throat and drippy nose. Clinically, I have found the pollen does not have to come from local sources to work. The two brands I use most often are Nature's Way® and Glory Bee®. Make sure it is pure bee pollen and does not contain addded ginseng.
- ❖ **Chinese Herbs**: For years I have managed the bulk of my allergy symptoms with Chinese herb teas. Now, I won't lie to you and say the stuff tastes great—it doesn't—but it works and I only have to drink between 4-8 ounces daily to keep my lungs happy and my head clear.
- ❖ **Bioflavonoid Complex** from Complimentary Prescription: This is nature's Singular®; the combined benefits of this product benefit blood pressure, circulation, heart health and the combination of bioflavonoids work as a mast cell inhibitor. I have tried dozens of similar products from other companies, and always end up going back to the product from VRP because it consistently performs well for all ages.
- ❖ **OPC** or grape seed extract: All of the antioxidants, including vitamins C and E, play an important role in the reduction of inflammation. As we have seen, allergies are a form of inflammation and they respond well to antioxidants. OPC stands for *Oligomeric Proanthocyanidin*, a very powerful antioxidant found in grape seed and a truckload of other foods. As with all natural health options, synergistic combinations require lower doses and provide more bang for your dollar.

With all of these protocols, you will have to take more than one every 24 hours. But the benefits far outweigh the inconvenience of taking these nutraceuticals several times daily.

Some individuals are highly sensitive to fungus in the forms of both mushrooms and mold. Mold sickness and exposure-related illnesses are significant. Mold has been linked to lung damage, brain damage, cancer and even death. The recent discovery of "Mold Fine Particulates" in our environment coupled with the associated medical documentation prove sickness from mold exposure is very real.

If mold spores are inhaled or ingested you can become severely ill. As the mold continues to grow inside your body it produces poisons called mycotoxins; these poisons leach into your body day after day. Every day the colonies of mold grow larger, producing and releasing larger amounts of toxins into your body.

Different species of mold produce different toxins and people will suffer a wide range of symptoms.

Because the variety of symptoms from mold exposure are so broad in range, many physicians decide that their patients simply have psychological problems.
The most commonly reported symptoms of short-term mold exposure:

Sneezing	Watery Eyes
Itching Skin	Redness and Skin Irritation
Itching Eyes	

HeadacheThe following symptoms of mold exposure have been reported generally as a result from persons being in a mold-contaminated environment on and off for an extended period of time. Symptoms are reported to have become more severe and longer lasting directly in proportion to the length of exposure time.
Their reported symptoms are:

Constant headaches	Neurological & nervous disorders
Nose bleeds	Sexual dysfunction
Feelings of constant fatigue	Swollen glands in the neck area and
Breathing disorders	armpit
Coughing up blood or black looking	Sudden asthma attacks or breathing
debris	disorders
Nausea	Ear infections and pain
Diarrhea	Chronic sinus infections
Vomiting	Chronic bronchitis
Loss of appetite	Pain in the joints and muscle[136]
Weight loss	
Hair loss	
Skin rashes	
Open sores on the skin	
Memory loss, short-term	

---

[136] Mold Symptoms.Org - Developed For the Public's Better Understanding of The Dangers Of Fungal Contamination and Infections

Severe reactions may occur among workers exposed to large amounts of molds in occupational settings, such as farmers working around moldy hay or in greenhouses. Severe reactions may include fever and shortness of breath. Immunocompromised persons and persons with chronic lung diseases like COPD are at increased risk for opportunistic infections and may develop fungal infections in their lungs.

In 2004, the *Institute of Medicine* (IOM) found there was sufficient evidence to link indoor exposure to mold with upper respiratory tract symptoms, coughing and wheezing in otherwise healthy people; with asthma symptoms in people with asthma; and with hypersensitivity pneumonitis in individuals susceptible to that immune-mediated condition. The IOM also found limited or suggestive evidence linking indoor mold exposure and respiratory illness in otherwise healthy children.

This is yet another reason to eat immune-supporting foods like onion, garlic, oregano, basil and rosemary while limiting the consumption of the toxic foods found in the modern American diet.[137,138]

---

[137] http://www.cdc.gov/mold/stachy.htm
[138] http://www.biosignlabs.com/Symptoms_Mold_Sickness.html

In 2011, the FDA began the process of approving a genetically modified salmon for human consumption. They said that at this time they have no reason to believe it is harmful to humans. But what happens if these modified fish escape their hatchery nets, like fish often do, and breed with wild salmon? Fish in these farming environments already escape into the wild by the millions every year. What are the potential ramifications to the ecosystem, aqua businesses and the species as a whole? If approved, the genetically modified (GM) salmon—known as AquAdvantage—will be the first GM animal officially authorized for human consumption in the U.S.

Aqua Bounty Technologies Inc.®, the company responsible for the new salmon, has been seeking approval from the FDA since 1995. By programming salmon genes to continuously produce growth hormone, scientists from the company have been able to make their engineered fish grow to full size in less than 250 days, as opposed to the 400 days it takes for a natural Atlantic salmon to grow. Aqua Bounty® researchers have told the FDA the production of GM fish will improve the fish economy and reduce environmental stress.

The company claims that the fish are sterile, pose no environmental or health threats and taste like real fish, but not everyone is convinced. Previous studies have shown the opposite to be true. In 1999, researchers from Purdue University found transgenic fish are more attractive to other fish because of their abnormally large size. So they beat out real fish in attracting breeding mates, which can cause serious problems if introduced into the wild.

The same study also found the offspring of transgenic fish live very short lives. According to the university report, 60 fertile GM fish placed in a population of 60,000 native fish could destroy the entire native stock in as little as 20 years. Despite claims this could never occur because the fish are sterile, many experts say the DNA in GM fish will mutate over time and cause them to be able to breed. They could then spread their DNA to other species, altering the genetic makeup of fish everywhere.

Let me first point out that Atlantic salmon is not a true salmon and the food quality of this seagoing trout, what we in the west call steelhead, is inferior to Alaskan, British Canadian and Pacific Northwest salmon (Coho, King, Chinook or Sockeye).

These fish live in the ocean for 7 years and only return to the inland streams when it is time to breed, and die. While they are living in the ocean they are living on shrimp, krill and smaller fish, not the standard fish hatchery and farm food fare of soy, corn, wheat and protein by-products.

Atlantic salmon are also exposed to significant quantities of toxins from runoff water in the eastern United States. The potentially high levels of mercury, lead, cadmium, arsenic, PCBs and prescription medications not only affect the overall health of the fish but the health of those who consume them. One more strike against farm-raised Atlantic salmon is the balance of omega-3 to omega-6 oil. This ratio is off due to the differences in the diet of wild fish versus farmed. Wild fish is naturally high in omega-3 oils, which have been found to prevent heart disease, diabetes, depression and inflammation. Corn, soy and grains elevate omega-6 levels in the fish, reducing its health benefits and driving inflammation as excess omega-6 converts into prostaglandin 2, a precursor of degenerative illness.

I won't delve into the environmental impact of farm-raised fish, but know that it is considerable and affects water, soils and oceanic health.

According to a recent *Reuters* article, the FDA has failed to release any of the safety data about Aqua Bounty's® GM fish, so nobody can say for sure what its potential health effects would be. But concerned groups say that, like other GM foods, AquAdvantage fish may cause allergies, digestive problems and other serious illness. "To date, there have been no studies conducted proving that any GM foods are safe for human consumption. And the studies that have been carried out show that tampering with nature at the genetic level only causes problems for people and the environment, not benefits," stated Dr. Michael Antoniou, a British molecular scientist.[139]

For centuries, politicians and world leaders have used food sources to manipulate populations, leading to widespread famine and population control. History buffs should check out the book *Taste of War* by Lizzie Collingham.

We are at a crossroads in history. For the first time we have gone from selective breeding and hybridization to genetic engineering. This has been done because of the belief that "we can feed the world through science." The most impressive advance in agriculture was the advent of fertilizer that allowed for more nitrogen to be available than what was naturally occurring in nature. This advance allowed for more to be fed from smaller areas of land; that is until the soil degraded too far to

---

[139] The GMO Deception 2014

support a burgeoning population. Pushing the soil too far can be a slippery slope; the Dust Bowl is one example of the consequences. Patrick Allitt recounts how fellow historian Donald Worster responded to his return visit to the Dust Bowl in the mid-1970s when he revisited some of the worst afflicted counties:

"Capital-intensive agribusiness had transformed the scene; deep wells into the aquifer, intensive irrigation, the use of artificial pesticides and fertilizers, and giant harvesters were creating immense crops year after year whether it rained or not. According to the farmers he interviewed, technology had provided the perfect answer to old troubles, such of the bad days would not return. In Worster's view, by contrast, the scene demonstrated that America's capitalist high-tech farmers had learned nothing. They were continuing to work in an unsustainable way, devoting far cheaper subsidized energy to growing food than the energy could give back to its ultimate consumers." (Patrick Allitt, A Climate of Crisis: America in the Age of Environmentalism (2014) p 203)

Today many states are doing battle over GMO food labeling, and not over their development, sale or use. I personally believe I have the right to make food purchases based on my beliefs; one is that I like to buy local produce to keep more of my money in the local economy. I also believe it is wrong to manipulate DNA and RNA for profit.

Have You Ever Really Asked The Question "What is Food?"

When I ask, "What is food?" I hear answers like "It is something that gives you

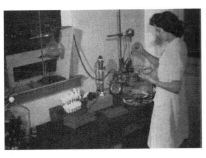

energy and something you eat and cook." I also hear, "Pizza, french fries, hamburgers, macaroni and cheese, ice cream, burrito, chips, hot dogs," and sometimes, "apples." Technically this is all true. The formal definition is: "material consisting essentially of protein, carbohydrate and fat used in the body of an organism to sustain growth, repair vital processes and to furnish energy; also, something that nourishes, sustains, or supplies nutriment in solid form."[140]

When I ask myself this question, the words that come to mind are: culture, economy, stability, politics, industry, science, freedom and health.

---

[140] Websters Dictionary

Let me explain: "Better living through science" was all the rage in the 1940s and 1950s. The food industry became dominated by this world view.

When a grain crop in Oregon (2013) or Montana (2014) is contaminated by GMOs, the cost isn't as small as you might think. "Genetically engineered wheat has surfaced at a second unauthorized location in the U.S.," the Agriculture Department said, raising new questions about agricultural companies' oversight of biotech crops. On September 26, 2014, the USDA said "that it began an investigation into genetically engineered plants discovered in July at Montana State University's Southern Agricultural Research Center." The finding came as the USDA closed its investigation into the detection of genetically engineered wheat in Oregon in 2013. *(Wall Street Journal)(USDA News Releases)*

Each time these little "mistakes" happen, the economic ripple doesn't stop with the farmers losing their high-value export contracts to Russia, China, Japan, South Korea and so forth. Nor does it necessarily benefit Canada, who competes for these same grain export contracts. When I think about all the jobs and businesses impacted, I see shipping companies, truck drivers, repair shops, lawyers, commodity brokers, advertisers, equipment manufacturers, fuel companies, retailers, state and county coffers, and more. Jobs and lifestyles are so interwoven with food we forget just how many folks a farmer actually feeds. The unforeseen consequences reach far beyond manufacturing labels and personal health.

Food isn't just a piece of fruit, a slab of sirloin steak or a slice of artisan bread that we smack our lips over, it is what fuels our creativity, independence, intellect and civilization. Our food makes or breaks our empire, just as it did the Romans, Mesopotamians and Stalin's armies. I'm all for science, but I would prefer to not be the research lab rat, and I don't want the next generation used as one either. Biotech foods may be the answer to world hunger or population control, they may revolutionize agriculture or destroy it; GMOs have only been in our food supply for a decade. How long did it take for the dangers of Agent Orange or DDT to be realized?

Looking More At The Environmental Issues.

While some may feel this is a small issue, I ask you to reconsider. What happens when squash, tomatoes and potatoes from GE sources cross-contaminate non-GE crops? How do you feel about receiving your vaccines through your potatoes? Won't happen, the experts say. And I have a bridge for sale...

In fact, this has already happened. The loss of native, heirloom and, most importantly, fertile food crops will be devastating to local economies, food stores, populations and health. The potato was converted into a vehicle for the cholera vaccine; they are working out the kinks in transportation methods now. Tomatoes were engineered to carry antibiotics and the FDA halted sales, but it is being revisited; GE squash fled the field along with rice quickly after its first planting.

"Government scientists have stated that the artificial insertion of DNA into plants, a technique unique to genetic engineering, can cause a variety of significant problems with plant foods. Such genetic engineering can increase the levels of known toxicants in foods and introduce new toxicants and health concerns.

"... Genetic engineering of plants and animals often causes unintended consequences. Manipulating genes and inserting them into organisms is an imprecise process. The results are not always predictable or controllable, and they can lead to adverse health or environmental consequences/

"... Fifty countries—including the European Union member states, Japan and other key U.S. trading partners—have laws mandating disclosure of genetically engineered foods. No international agreements prohibit the mandatory identification of foods produced through genetic engineering."[141]

In addition, 26 years of research and 19 years of commercialization reveal that GE has failed to significantly increase U.S. crop yields. Instead, it has resulted in farmers having to buy more pesticides and increased the prices on patented seeds.

Current FDA policy is that genetically engineered foods do not need to be labeled, arguing genetically engineered foods are "substantially equivalent" to non-GE foods.[142, 143, 144, 145]

On March 14, 2014, Kroger and Safeway, the largest retail grocery companies in the U.S., announced their decision to not sell genetically modified salmon. The two grocery chains are now part of more than 9,000 stores across the country that have rejected carrying the GM AquAdvantage® salmon regardless of whether the U.S.

---

[141] www.anh-usa.org/stop-monsanto-rider-in-senate/

[142] www.webmd.com/food-recipes/features/are-biotech-foods-safe-to-eat

[143] www.nationalhealthfreedom.org/nhfa/Alerts/14StateActionNeeded_031513.htm#states

[144] www.anh-usa.org/stop-monsanto-rider-in-senate/

[145] www.fda.gov/animalveterinary/developmentapprovalprocess/geneticengineering/geneticallyengineeredanimals/ucm113672.htm

Food and Drug Administration approves it for public consumption, which it has not yet officially done.[146]

Call me old-fashioned, but I think nature has done a pretty great job of making living organisms. I'm not convinced we can do a better job. By the way, the FDA will not be requiring the manufacturers to label their salmon product as a GM food—you the consumer will have no idea that what you are eating has been genetically altered.

What will our DNA think of this food? We already know our DNA looks for specific links to tie into for healthy replication. Will GM foods fail to meet our DNA's needs and increase the rates of cancer, hereditary diseases and premature aging? I don't know, and I'm not willing to risk it.

---

[146] www.foodsafetynews.com/2014/03/kroger-safeway-turn-down-gmo-salmon-regardless-of-fda/#.U6HtQCiGff4

Type 2 diabetes is so common, it is assumed by many that they will "get it" like a cold or flu bug as they get older. The truth of the matter is, type 2 diabetes is one of the most preventable illnesses. It is largely unique to industrialized countries and is directly caused by diet and lifestyle. "My grandfather had diabetes," a client will say to me. I ask, "How old was your grandfather when he was diagnosed with diabetes?" "Oh, he was in his late seventies." As we age our cells become more resistant to insulin and sugars. This is in large part due to the lack of exercise many older (and today's younger folks) are getting. And the foods most often eaten by older people are those highest in sugar forming content—carbohydrates.

My mother came from southern stock. Cornbread soaked in sweet milk or buttermilk was a favorite. The problem is that her blood sugars would go through the roof because her blood stream was unable to process all the sugar formed by these foods. Today's version may be saltine crackers, chips or snack cookies. I have learned through clinical research that three saltine crackers will elevate my clients' blood sugars faster than glucose tabs or gel—good to know if you are traveling with a type 1 diabetic.

It is important to know that new technology has enabled scientists to prove that most people with type 1 diabetes have active beta cells, the specialized insulin-making cells found in the pancreas. Type 1 diabetes occurs when the body's immune system destroys the cells making insulin, the substance that enables glucose in the blood to gain access to the body's cells.

It was previously thought that all of these cells were lost within a few years of developing the condition. However, new research led by the University of Exeter Medical School, which has been funded by Diabetes UK and published in *Diabetologia* (the journal of the European Association for the Study of Diabetes), shows that around three-quarters of patients with the condition possess a small number of beta cells that are not only producing insulin, but are producing it in response to food in the same way as someone without the condition.[147]

Sixty percent of the glucose converted from our food goes straight to feed the brain; the rest is used for rapid energy or put into fat storage. The foods we eat and drink

---

[147] Diabetologia. "Insulin 'still produced' in most people with type 1 diabetes." ScienceDaily. ScienceDaily, 9 October 2013. <www.sciencedaily.com/releases/2013/10/131009213816.htm>.

have a direct and profound effect on our brain; the brain is the central computer that controls the rest of the body's chemical responses.

The "SAD" (Standard American Diet) is loaded with foodstuffs that the digestive system breaks down into sugar—a lot of sugar. Highly refined flour, found in crackers, bread, TV dinners, coating mixes, cereals and fast foods, are the worst. When you combine all the GMO fats (canola oil) and sugars (high fructose corn syrup) with these grain products the liver goes into a tailspin and the pancreas cries out for help. Cholesterols, blood sugars and insulin climb, affecting blood pressure, heart health, liver health and cognition.

What To Do?

It may not be reasonable to expect everyone to give up their favorite restaurant, but if Americans are going to get healthy it will not be because of a new health care bill, drug or insurance company. It will be because the populace started being proactive about healthy eating, nutrient supplementation, exercise and stress management.

Eat locally grown meat and eggs—organic or home-raised. Consume three to five ounces of protein per meal or about 30 grams per day. Look at the palm of your hand—that is about how much real meat you need per meal.

Start your meal with raw or steamed vegetables and a tablespoon of vinegar—no potatoes, and iceberg lettuce doesn't count. The darker the greens, the better for your liver and eyes. Raw carrots and snap peas make great snacks but if cooked they are prone to elevating blood sugars.

Cooking with olive oil, unrefined coconut oil, organic butter, walnut oil and macadamia nut oil make blood sugars more stable. The additional health benefits of these oils protect nerves from damage.[148]

According to a study released in 2014, the diabetes rate in the United States has nearly doubled in the past 10 years. Approximately 26 million Americans are now classified as diabetic, stressing an urgent need for safe and effective complementary strategies to enhance the existing conventional treatment for diabetes. Preliminary studies have demonstrated that grape skin extract (GSE) exerts a novel inhibitory activity on hyperglycemia and could be developed and used to aid in diabetes management.

---

[148] (Daniella Chace, 1998)

With type 2 diabetes, the body does not produce enough insulin or the cells ignore the insulin. Some population groups have a higher risk of developing type 2 diabetes, including African Americans, Latinos, Native Americans, Asian Americans/Pacific Islanders and the elderly.

A 2014 study by researchers at the Harvard School of Public Health found that those who improved their diet quality index scores by 10 percent over four years (by eating more whole grains, fruits and vegetables, and less sweetened beverages and saturated fats, for example) reduced their risk for type 2 diabetes by about 20 percent, compared to those who made no changes to their diets.[149]

"It threatens the health of a variety of populations, with growing numbers of young people being diagnosed with the disease every day. Dr. Zhou's study offers great hope for a potential treatment that is natural and without harmful side effects for the many people with type 2 diabetes," the study from Wayne State University Division of Research reported.[150]

Fasting & Diabetes

Fasting is often overlooked as a method of preventing chronic diseases such as diabetes. The Mediterranean diet and Blue Zones® both note that fasting, as practiced in various cultures, can help prevent diabetes and heart disease.

At the Intermountain Heart Institute at Intermountain Medical Center in Murray, Utah, researchers noticed that after 10 to 12 hours of fasting, the body starts scavenging for other sources of energy to sustain itself. The body pulls LDL (bad) cholesterol from the fat cells and uses it for energy.

"Fasting has the potential to become an important diabetes intervention," says Benjamin Horne, PhD, director of cardiovascular and genetic epidemiology at the Intermountain Medical Center Heart Institute and lead researcher on the study. "Though we've studied fasting and it's health benefits for years, we didn't know why fasting could provide the health benefits we observed related to the risk of diabetes."[151]

---

[149] American Diabetes Association. "Improving diet quality reduces risk for type 2 diabetes." ScienceDaily. ScienceDaily, 14 June 2014. <www.sciencedaily.com/releases/2014/06/140614150313.htm>.

[150] Wayne State University Division of Research. "Grape skin extract may soon be answer to treating diabetes." ScienceDaily. ScienceDaily, 9 May 2014. <www.sciencedaily.com/releases/2014/05/140509110201.htm>.

[151] Intermountain Medical Center. "Fasting reduces cholesterol levels in prediabetic people over extended period of time, new research finds." ScienceDaily. ScienceDaily, 14 June 2014. <www.sciencedaily.com/releases/2014/06/140614150142.htm>.

This is the first evidence of a natural intervention triggering stem cell-based regeneration of an organ or system. It shows that cycles of prolonged fasting not only protect against immune system damage—a major side effect of chemotherapy—but also induce immune system regeneration, shifting stem cells from a dormant state to a state of self-renewal.[152]

Maybe religious traditions like fasting are good for the body as well as the mind and soul?

Supplements Are a Must

> ➤ Chromium and vanadium are found to be deficient in diabetics. They play a significant role in blood sugar regulation and uptake into the cells.
> ➤ Selenium is an antioxidant and necessary for healthy cell formation.
> ➤ Vitamin C is a daily must: 2000 mg daily for protecting cells, blood sugar regulation and heart health.
> ➤ Remember, heart disease and diabetes go hand in hand. Avoid the ascorbic acid form of vitamin C as it is manufactured primarily in China and is heavily contaminated with heavy metals.
> ➤ B-complex vitamins are a daily requirement. It is important to protect the brain and nervous system from damage. B vitamins play a vital role in keeping the entire body healthy.
> ➤ Antioxidants from OPC (*Oligomeric Proanthocyanidins*)and resveratrol.
> ➤ Probiotics for healthy gut bacteria are the superstars in correcting, maintaining and balancing digestive health when it comes to the breakdown of carbohydrates. When our digestion is slow, sluggish or overactive, our blood sugars are profoundly affected. These beneficial bacteria are proving to be our health's best friends.
> ➤ There are several herbal products that help to stabilize sugar cravings. I have found a MediHerb product called Gymnema.[153] This product was first recommended to me by an herbalist, and then later by Dianna Schwasbein, MD.
> ➤ Last but not least, exercise. Modern life has made physical movement a chore for many. No longer are we walking to and fro feeding animals, working in the garden or fields, climbing stairs, or walking to the bakery and butcher. All of this movement that was just a normal part of life was

[152] University of Southern California. "Fasting triggers stem cell regeneration of damaged, old immune system." ScienceDaily. ScienceDaily, 5 June 2014.
www.sciencedaily.com/releases/2014/06/140605141507.htm.
[153] Standard Process Fundamentals – MediHerb (800)292-6699

instrumental in helping those heartier foods we crave like potatoes, breads, pastas, rice, beets and winter squash to better metabolize.

Mild weight-lifting and strength-building exercises should be done at least three times a week to maintain bone health, circulation, brain health and balance. People who live in neighborhoods that are conducive to walking experience a substantially lower rate of obesity and diabetes than those who lived in more auto-dependent neighborhoods, according to a pair of studies.

Specifically, the studies found that people living in neighborhoods with greater "walkability" saw on average a 13% lower development of diabetes incidence over ten years than those that were less walkable.[154] For many individuals, physical therapy is the best place to start. Therapists will help you establish a workout program that is appropriate for your abilities. They can help you stay motivated and keep you from having injuries that would cut short your efforts.

---

[154] American Diabetes Association. "Do 'walkable' neighborhoods reduce obesity, diabetes? Yes, research suggests." ScienceDaily. ScienceDaily, 17 June 2014. <www.sciencedaily.com/releases/2014/06/140617130824.htm>.

Vitamin A

In his book *Eat and Be Healthy,* published in 1919, Virgil MacMickle, MD, of Portland, Oregon, recognized how crucial nutrition was to health. He wrote that the "chemical substances of which the body is composed are very similar to those of the foods which nourish it. They are made up of the same chemical elements. ...The body can only get the materials from which it is made in the first place from foods."

There are 13 known vitamins, of which four are fat-soluble; the remaining nine are water-soluble. A fat-soluble vitamin is absorbed with the help of fat. Vitamins A, D, E and K are fat-soluble.

A Little History

Three thousand five hundred years ago, the ancient Egyptians recognized that night blindness (caused by a lack of vitamin A) could be treated with particular foods. Native Alaskan Indians made a point of eating the eyes of the fish and animals they hunted, believing they would keep the eyes of the hunter and his family healthy.

In 1913, attention turned to finding and isolating the vitamins themselves. The actual discovery of vitamin A is credited to a researcher named E. V. McCollum. He was curious as to why cows fed wheat did not thrive, became blind and gave birth to dead calves, while those fed yellow corn had no health problems. Thomas Osborne and Lafayette Mendel showed in rat experiments conducted at Yale University that butter contained a growth-promoting factor necessary for development. Soon known as fat-soluble vitamin A, its chemical character was established in 1933, and it was synthesized in 1947. Weston A. Price discovered the diets of healthy traditional peoples contained at least ten times as much vitamin A as the American diet of his day (1939). Weston Price's work revealed vitamin A is one of several fat-soluble activators present only in animal fats and necessary for the assimilation of minerals in the diet.

More Than Your Eyes

Many have been led to believe that the best way to get vitamin A is via beta-carotene. While it is true that many vegetables are loaded with health-promoting carotenoids, not everyone can increase or correct a vitamin A deficiency with plant-based foods. There are several factors that could potentially interfere with the conversion of carotenes in plant foods to vitamin A, such as being an infant or child, eating a low-fat diet, or having a condition like diabetes, low thyroid function, diarrhea, celiac disease, gluten sensitivity or pancreatic disease.

Naturally occurring vitamin A is necessary for the prevention of anemia (due to vitamin A enhancing the absorption of iron), heart disease, blood clots, stroke, hemorrhoids, loss of appetite, celiac disease, colitis, Crohn's disease, heartburn, peptic ulcers, ulcerative colitis, deafness, tinnitus, urinary tract infections, macular degeneration, blurred vision, dry eye and more.

The Merck Manual describes vitamin A toxicity as follows: "Acute vitamin A poisoning can occur in children after taking a single dose of "synthetic" vitamin A in the range of 300,000 IU or a daily dosage of 60,000 IU for a few weeks. In adults, vitamin A toxicity has been reported in Arctic explorers who developed drowsiness, irritability, headaches and vomiting, with subsequent peeling of the skin, within a few hours of ingesting several million units of vitamin A, from polar bear or seal liver. Symptoms cleared up with discontinuation of the vitamin A rich food. Vitamin A toxicity is much more common with the use of megavitamin tablets containing synthetic vitamin A. Acute toxicity occures at, 100,000 IU synthetic vitamin A, per day taken for many months."

Listed are approximate levels of vitamin A in common foods, in IUs per 100 grams:

- High-vitamin cod liver oil: 230,000
- Regular cod liver oil: 100,000
- Duck liver: 40,000
- Beef liver: 35,000
- Goose liver: 31,000
- Liverwurst sausage (pork): 28,000
- Lamb liver: 25,000

It should be noted that these amounts can vary according to how the animals are fed.

The U.S. Recommended Daily Allowance of vitamin A is currently 5,000 IU per day. From the work of Weston A. Price, we know the amount in primitive diets was about 50,000 IU per day. If you consume generous quantities of raw whole milk, cream, butter and eggs from pastured animals; beef or duck liver several times per week;

and 1 tablespoon regular cod liver oil or 1/2 tablespoon high-vitamin cod liver oil per day, you can come close to that.

Some individuals may choose to supplement instead. If you do, make sure you find a reputable brand, and know that top-quality comes with a hefty price. If you like liver, contact a local farmer who raises grass-fed animals.

"B" To The Rescue

Seemingly every day in my office, clients talk about how tired they are, how their brains are not working, how they are under so much stress and how their health seems to be slipping away. Some of these clients have a long history of chronic illness and nutritional deficiencies. Others are young, even adolescent, and they are tired, listless and depressed.

How can a country with so many resources have so many sick citizens? Every day we consume thousands of calories—calories without the nutrients.

Being healthy is about more than just calories; it involves a complex and synergistic balance of nutrients. Have we ever been able to get everything we need from our food? For today's modern man, my answer is no; it is not physically possible for us to obtain enough nutrients from food without bursting from the mountain of food required. But today we can supplement.

On May 19, 2014, a research study on B vitamins and how they help prevent childhood asthma was published:

> *"Maternal intake of dietary methyl donors during the first trimester of pregnancy modulates the risk of developing childhood asthma at age 7, according to a new study presented at the 2014 American Thoracic Society International Conference.*
>
> *'Evidence on the effects of dietary methyl donor intake on childhood asthma has been mixed,' said lead author Michelle Trivedi, MD, Clinical Fellow in Pediatric Pulmonology at Massachusetts General Hospital for Children in Boston. 'It has been suggested that folate enrichment of some foods may have contributed to the increasing asthma and allergy prevalence in the U.S. In our study of more than 1,000 mother-child pairs, we found that maternal intake of the six methyl donors we studied, folate, choline, betaine, and vitamins B2, B6 and B12, had protective effects on the risk of developing childhood asthma,*

and that interactions between these nutrients affected the magnitude and the direction of this risk.'

Methyl donors are nutrients involved in a biochemical process called methylation, in which chemicals are linked to proteins, DNA, or other molecules in the body. This process is involved in a number of important functions in the body, and dietary intake of methyl donors has been shown to affect the risk of developing a number of diseases, including heart disease and cancer."[155]

When we look at the history of food and how it has affected the civilizations of the world, we see some rather startling trends. Trends just as prevalent today as in the time of the Romans, Greeks, Mayans, and ancient India and China:

- When a civilization can no longer feed its citizens, it begins to crumble.
- When the land can no longer produce enough food to feed the populace, the populace migrates.
- When the food has no nutritional value the populace becomes ill, cannibalism occurs and the population/culture dies off.

If this sounds harsh or extremist to you, I encourage you to read Reay Tannahill's book *Food in History* from Three Rivers Press.

So what does this have to do with B vitamins? B vitamins were the first nutrients to be recognized as vital to health. Rarely are B vitamins found in singles; they are found in complex groupings within foods. The synergy of these groupings reduces the likelihood of deficiencies from over-consumption of a single B vitamin. Chinese physicians wrote about thiamin (B1) in the early 7th century. The Japanese and later the Europeans learned that animals became ill when fed refined grains.

Thiamin (B1) is a water-soluble B-complex vitamin. It was the first B vitamin to be identified and one of the first organic compounds to be recognized as a vitamin in the 1930s. It was through this discovery and naming of thiamin that the word *vitamine* from the Latin "vita" (life) and "amine" (nitrogen-containing compound) was coined. The notion that the absence of a substance in food could cause a disease (beriberi) was a revolutionary one.

---

[155] American Thoracic Society. "Intake of dietary methyl donors in first trimester affects asthma risk in children." ScienceDaily. ScienceDaily, 19 May 2014.
<www.sciencedaily.com/releases/2014/05/140519184542.htm>.

A Little History

I find it fascinating that we have a long tradition of studying nutrients, one that the FDA, AMA and pharmaceutical companies ignore in favor of designer drugs.

- 7th century: First classical description of beriberi in a *General Treatise on the Etiology and Symptoms of Diseases* by Ch'ao-Yuan-fang Wu Ching.
- 1882: Kanehiro Takaki, Navy Surgeon General, dramatically decreases the incidence of beriberi in the Japanese navy by improving sailors' diets.
- 1897: Dutch medical officers Eijkman and Grijns show that the symptoms of beriberi can be reproduced in chickens fed on polished rice, and that these symptoms can be prevented or cured by feeding them rice bran.
- 1937: The first commercial production of thiamin is accomplished.
- 1943: Williams and coworkers, and Foltz and colleagues carry out dietary studies that document widespread thiamin deficiency in the United States.
- 1943: Standards of identity for enriched flour are created by the U.S. Food and Nutrition Board, requiring that thiamin, niacin, riboflavin and iron be added to white flour.

B1 Main Functions

- Co-enzyme in energy metabolism; B1 is an essential compound for several reactions in the breakdown of glucose to energy
- Co-enzyme for pentose metabolism as a basis for nucleic acids
- Nerve impulse conduction and muscle action

Thiamin (B1) is found in small amounts in most foods. The best sources are dried brewer's yeast, meat (especially pork, eel and tuna), whole grain cereals and bread, nuts, dried legumes and potatoes.

The thiamin-rich bran is removed during milling of wheat to produce white flour, and during the polishing of brown rice to produce white rice. As a consequence, synthetically enriched and fortified grain products are the standard fare today.

Absorption of B1 occurs in the small intestine. Because thiamin has a high turnover rate and is not appreciably stored in the body, regular intake of B1 is critical. The limited stores are depleted within two weeks or less; clinical signs of deficiency begin shortly after. The heart, kidney, liver and brain have the highest concentrations, followed by the leukocytes and red blood cells.

The presence of other B vitamins such as vitamins B6, B12, niacin and pantothenic acid supports the action of thiamin. Antioxidant vitamins, such as vitamins E and C, protect thiamin by preventing oxidation.

Foods such as coffee, tea, betel nuts (Southeast Asia) and some cereals act as antagonists to thiamin. Drugs that cause nausea and lack of appetite, or which increase intestinal function or urinary excretion, decrease the availability of thiamin. Poisoning from arsenic or other heavy metals produces the neurological symptoms of thiamin deficiency. Marginal thiamin deficiency may manifest in vague symptoms such as fatigue, insomnia, irritability, lack of concentration, anorexia, abdominal discomfort, constipation and loss of appetite. When there is not enough B1, the overall decrease in carbohydrate metabolism and its interconnection with amino acid metabolism has severe consequences.

Causes of Deficiency

➢ Alcoholic disease
➢ Inadequate storage and preparation of food
➢ Increased demand due to pregnancy and lactation, heavy physical exertion, fever and stress, or adolescent growth
➢ Inadequate nutrition
➢ High carbohydrate intake (milled or polished rice, sweets)
➢ Regular consumption of tea and coffee
➢ Regular consumption of raw fish or betel nuts
➢ Certain diseases (dysentery, diarrhea, cancer, nausea/vomiting, liver diseases, infections, malaria, AIDS, hyperthyroidism)
➢ Drugs (birth-control pills, neuroleptica, some cancer drugs)
➢ Long-term parenteral nutrition (e.g. highly concentrated dextrose infusions)

Riboflavin (B2)

Riboflavin (B2) is one of the most widely distributed water-soluble vitamins. B2 can be isolated from milk, eggs, liver, plants and urine. The term "flavin" originates from the Latin word "flavus" referring to the yellow color of this vitamin. The fluorescent riboflavin is a part of B-complex vitamins, and is the cause of bright yellow urine after taking multivitamins or B-complexes.

As with all B vitamins, B2 must be replaced in the body each and every day. All processed foods have riboflavin listed on the label, as well as fortified flour and cereal foods. However heat, light and processing destroys B vitamins, so the nutritional value of processed foods is questionable.

Riboflavin is an essential constituent of all living cells. However, there are very few foods that contain significant quantities. Yeast and liver have the highest concentrations, but are not usually part of the standard American diet. The most common dietary sources are (organic) milk and dairy products, lean meat, eggs and green leafy vegetables. Cereal grains are inferior sources of riboflavin. Animal sources of riboflavin are absorbed at the highest rate and are better than vegetable sources. In milk from cows, sheep and goats, at least 90% of the riboflavin is in the "free" form, making it immediately available to the body. Because B2 is degraded by light, up to 50% may be lost if foods are left out in sunlight or under UV light (85% within 2 hours).

History of B Vitamin Isolation. (*History of Vitamin B2 - davidfood. (n.d.). Retrieved from http://davidfood.over-blog.com/article-history-of-vitamin-b2-103154727.html_br)*

1879   Blyth isolates lactochrome, a water-soluble, yellow fluorescent material, from whey.

1932   Warburg and Christian extract a yellow enzyme from brewer's yeast and suggest that it plays an important part in cell respiration.

1933   Kuhn and coworkers obtain a crystalline yellow pigment with growth-promoting properties from egg white and whey, which they identify as vitamin B2.

1934   Kuhn and associates in Heidelberg, and Karrer and colleagues in Zurich, synthesize pure riboflavin.

1937   The Council on Pharmacy and Chemistry of the American Medical Association names the vitamin "riboflavin".

1941   Sebrell and coworkers demonstrate clinical signs of riboflavin deficiency in human feeding experiments.

Functions

- Energy production
- Antioxidant functions
- Conversion of vitamin B6 and folic acid into their active coenzyme forms
- Growth and reproduction
- Growth of skin, hair and nails
- Necessary to produce collagen
- Increases serum ferritin (an iron-storage protein)
- Cofactor in production of Superoxide Dismutase (SOD)
- Reduce the body's urinary excretion of selenium
- Lowers homocysteine levels

Clinically, vitamin B2 deficiency affects many organs and tissues. Most prominent are the effects on the skin, mucosa and eyes:

- ✓ magenta tongue, geographical tongue
- ✓ fissures at the corners of the mouth
- ✓ sore throat
- ✓ burning of the lips, mouth and tongue
- ✓ inflamed mucous membranes
- ✓ itching
- ✓ moist scaly skin inflammation
- ✓ corneal vascularization associated with sensitivity to bright light, impaired vision, itching and a feeling of grittiness in the eyes
- ✓ trauma, including burns and surgery
- ✓ chronic disorders (e.g. rheumatic fever, tuberculosis, subacute bacterial endocarditis, diabetes, hypothyroidism, liver cirrhosis)
- ✓ intestinal malabsorption, e.g. Crohn's disease, sprue, lactose intolerance
- ✓ chronic medication (tranquilizers, oral contraceptives, thyroid hormones, fiber-based laxatives, antibiotics)
- ✓ high physical activity
- ✓ phototherapy for newborns

Overt clinical symptoms of riboflavin deficiency are rarely seen in developed countries. However, subclinical deficiency is common. Riboflavin deficiency occurs in combination with deficiencies of other B-complex vitamins. Along with other B vitamins, low vitamin B2 levels have been associated with increased homocysteine levels and impaired absorption of iron, zinc and calcium.

Individuals at risk of deficiency are children from low socioeconomic backgrounds, the elderly, chronic dieters, addicts, people who are dairy-sensitive and vegans. Low riboflavin intake may be aggravated by chronic alcoholism and chronic stress; during pregnancy and lactation, riboflavin requirements increase.

With work, travel and life in general, it is very hard to avoid manufactured foods. But this is one reason why taking additional supplements are so important. We could all benefit from a good daily B-complex supplement.

Vitamin B6

In 2009, the FDA announced it was taking synthetic B6 off the market—not because of safety issues, but because it was so effective. Synthetic B6 (pyridoxamine) has been proven to be very effective in the treatment of neuropathy in diabetics. Because pyridoxamine is synthetically derived it can be placed under patent; this very inexpensive and efficient nutrient is about to join the ranks of controlled substances with designer drug pricing.

Humans and other primates depend on external sources to meet their vitamin B6 requirements. Vitamin B6 was discovered in the 1930s during the studies on pellagra, a deficiency disease caused by the absence in the body of the vitamin niacin. Negligible amounts of vitamin B6 can be synthesized by intestinal bacteria.

Main Functions

- ➤ Nervous system (neurotransmitter synthesis)
- ➤ Red blood cell formation
- ➤ Niacin formation
- ➤ Homocysteine down-regulation (preventing atherosclerosis)
- ➤ Immune system (antibody production)
- ➤ Steroid hormones (inhibition of the binding of steroid hormones)

Food Sources

Chicken and the liver of beef, pork and veal are excellent sources of B6 (pyridoxine). Good sources include fish (salmon, tuna, sardines, halibut and herring), nuts (walnuts and peanuts), bread, corn and whole grain cereals. Generally, vegetables and fruits are rather poor sources of vitamin B6, although there are three plant foods which contain considerable amounts of pyridoxine, such as lentils, courgettes (zucchini) and bananas.

Pasteurization causes milk to lose up to 20% of its vitamin B6 content. B6 is decomposed by oxidation and ultraviolet light, and by an alkaline environment. Because of this light sensitivity, vitamin B6 will disappear (50% within a few hours) from milk kept in glass bottles exposed to the sun or bright fluorescent light. Alkalis, such as baking soda, also destroy pyridoxine. Freezing of vegetables causes a reduction of up to 25%, while milling of cereals leads to losses as high as 90%. Cooking may result in losses ranging from a few percent to nearly half the vitamin B6 initially present.

B6 requires riboflavin, zinc and magnesium to fulfill its physiological function in humans. Women taking oral contraceptives have an increased requirement for B6 (pyridoxine). There are more than 40 drugs that interfere with vitamin B6, potentially causing decreased availability and inadequate vitamin B6 status.

B6 Toxicity in the Scotch and Irish

Enzymopathy of polymorphism of B6 is a genetic condition that is prevalent among people of Scotch and Irish decent where the enzyme that converts B6 into its useful form is too big. This causes excessive B6 to build up even if no supplement form is taken.[156],[157] This condition is being linked to neuropathy, ALS and MS. The restriction of all fortified grain products or B6 rich foods would be indicated for individuals testing high in B6 who are not using supplements. *Prevention & Therapeutic Use (Vitamin B6 - davidfood.* (n.d.). Retrieved from http://davidfood.over-blog.com/article-vitamin-b6-103216679.html_br)

1. Sideroblastic anemias and pyridoxine-dependent abnormalities of metabolism: B6 is an approved treatment for sideroblastic anemias and pyridoxine-dependent abnormalities of metabolism. In such cases, therapeutic doses of approximately 40-200 mg of vitamin B6 per day are indicated.
2. PMS (premenstrual syndrome): Studies suggest that vitamin B6 doses of up to 100 mg/day may help relieve the symptom complex of premenstrual syndrome.

---

[156] http://www.ncbi.nlm.nih.gov/pubmed/20056620
[157] Cancer Epidemiol Biomarkers Prev. 2010 Jan;19(1):28-38. doi: 10.1158/1055-9965.EPI-08-1096.

3. Hyperemesis gravidarum: Pyridoxine is often administered in doses of up to 40 mg/day in the treatment of nausea and vomiting during pregnancy (hyperemesis gravidarum).

4. Depression: B6 is used to assist in the relief of depression (especially in women taking oral contraceptives).

5. Carpal tunnel syndrome: Pyridoxine has been shown to alleviate the symptoms of carpal tunnel syndrome. However some studies report benefits while others do not.

6. Hyperhomocystinaemia/cardiovascular disease: Elevated homocysteine levels in the blood are considered a risk factor for atherosclerotic disease. Several studies have shown vitamin B6, vitamin B12 and folic acid can lower critical homocysteine levels.

7. Immune function: The elderly are a group that suffers from impaired immune function. Adequate B6 intake is important, and it has been shown that the amount of vitamin B6 required to improve the immune system is higher (2.4 mg/day for men; 1.9 mg/day for women) than the current RDA.

8. Asthma: Patients taking vitamin B6 supplements may have fewer and less severe attacks of wheezing, coughing and breathing difficulties.

9. Diabetes: Current research suggests patients with diabetes mellitus or gestational diabetes experience an improvement in glucose tolerance when given vitamin B6 supplements.

10. Kidney stones: Glyoxylate can be oxidized to oxalic acid that may lead to calcium oxalate kidney stones. Pyridoxal phosphate is a cofactor for the degradation of glyoxylate to glycine. There is evidence that high doses of vitamin B6 (>150 mg/day) are useful for normalizing the oxalic acid metabolism to reduce the formation of kidney stones.

11. "Chinese restaurant syndrome": People who are sensitive to glutamate, often used in the preparation of Asiatic dishes, can react with headache, tachycardia (accelerated heart rate) and nausea. Fifty to one hundred milligrams of pyridoxine can be of therapeutic value.

12. Autism: High-dose therapy with pyridoxine improves the status of autistics in about 30% of cases.

Vitamin B12

Vitamin B12 (cyanocobalamin) is commonly used as an injectable nutrient for those with anemia. Vitamin B12 is the largest and most complex of the vitamins. The term "vitamin B12" actually encompasses a particular group of cobalt-containing corrinoids biological activity in humans.[158] It is the only known metabolite to contain cobalt, which gives this water-soluble vitamin its red color.

The body's ability to absorb dietary vitamin B12 declines with the progression of the aging process (supplements of 500-1,000 micrograms per day are recommended to counteract impaired absorption in persons over the age of 60).

In 1934, three researchers won the Nobel Prize in medicine for discovering the lifesaving properties of vitamin B12. They found that eating large amounts of raw liver, which contains high amounts of vitamin B12, could save the life of previously incurable patients with pernicious anemia. This finding saves 10,000 lives a year in the U.S. alone. Vitamin B12 was isolated from liver extract in 1948 and its structure was elucidated 7 years later.

History

1926 Minot and Murphy report that a diet of large quantities of raw liver given to patients with pernicious anemia restores the normal level of red blood cells.

1948 Rickes and associates (U.S.) and Smith and Parker (England), isolate a crystalline red pigment which they name vitamin B12.

1948 West shows that injections of vitamin B12 dramatically benefit patients with pernicious anemia.

1955 Synthesis of vitamin B12 from cultures of certain bacteria/fungi.

1973 Total chemical synthesis of vitamin B12.

Functions

- Essential growth factor
- Formation of blood cells and nerve sheaths
- Prevent atherosclerosis and heart attacks
- Protect against the after-effects of (ischemic) stroke

---

[158] If my Vitamin B12 levels are above normal, is that OK? (n.d.). Retrieved from https://answers.yahoo.com/question/index?qid=20110224122408AAZugEJ_br

- Prevent damage to chromosomes
- Regeneration of folic acid
- Prevent neural tube defects
- Coenzyme-function in the intermediary metabolism, especially in cells of the nervous tissue, bone marrow and gastrointestinal tract[159]
- Enhance the general health of the digestive system
- Prevents cataracts
- Reverses the decline in mental function
- Treatment of hepatitis C
- Prevention of breast and lung cancer

Dietary Sources

Vitamin B12 is produced exclusively by microbial synthesis in the digestive tract of animals. Animal protein products are the best source of vitamin B12 in the human diet, in particular organ meats (liver, kidney). Other sources are fish, eggs and dairy products. Foods of plant origin contain no vitamin B12 beyond that derived from microbial contamination. Vitamin B12 from food sources is bound to proteins and is only released by an adequate concentration of hydrochloric acid in the stomach. In the human body, B12 content is found in the kidneys, heart, spleen and brain. B12 plasma concentrations peak at 8-12 hours after ingestion. Sublingual forms of B12 (methylcobalamin) have high absorption rates equal to injectable.
Absorption of B12 is impaired by alcohol, drug and vitamin B6 (pyridoxine) deficiency.

Supplementation May Be Necessary If Patient Has:
- Celiac disease
- Crohn's disease
- Chronic Fatigue Syndrome (CFS)
- 27% of people afflicted with chronic noise-induced hearing loss exhibit B12 deficiency
- 47% of tinnitus patients exhibit vitamin B12 deficiency

---

[159] Walpar Healthcare | Products - Healthcare. (n.d.). Retrieved from http://www.walpar.in/(S(e1pcm4ih5j155h45t5e1xnvd))/ayurvedic.html_br

May be needed when taking:
- Tuberculostatics
- Stomach medication: proton pump inhibitors, H2 receptor antagonists
- Liver medications
- Anti-gout medication
- Antibiotics
- Anti-diabetics: oral biguanides metformin and phenformin
- Potassium chloride medications
- Oral contraceptives
- Anticonvulsants
- Nitrous oxide (anesthetic) also interferes with B12 metabolism

Vitamin B12 deficiency occurs over several years, and is most obvious in vegetarians and vegans. Others with impaired digestion also have a reduced ability to absorb cobalamin via the intestine and develop a deficiency state more rapidly.

Best Form To Take

Methylcobalamin: active endogenous coenzyme form of vitamin B12 that transfers a methyl group from an inactive form of folic acid to homocysteine, forming methionine. This is the only active endogenous coenzyme form of vitamin B12. Methylcobalamin accounts for approximately 70% of the total blood plasma vitamin B12 reserves. Clinical trials have shown that supplemental methylcobalamin is substantially superior to other forms of vitamin B12 supplements in terms of its ability to enhance human health. The liver converts approximately 1% of the cyanocobalamin form of vitamin B12 to methylcobalamin.

Cyanocobalamin: complex of cyanide and cobalamin. This form of vitamin B12 is the most commonly found in vitamin B12 supplements. It must be converted to either of the active coenzyme forms within the body in order to exert therapeutic effects. It is not as effective as methylcobalamin. Most supplemental cyanocobalamin is converted within the intestines to adenosylcobalamin.

Niacin

Niacin is a member of the water-soluble B vitamin complex. The amino acid tryptophan can be converted to nicotinic acid in humans. Nicotinic acid is a specific form of vitamin B3. Nicotinic acid supplements are manufactured by oxidizing nicotine (this is not a cause for alarm as nicotinic acid is not associated with any of the toxic effects attributable to nicotine). Nicotinic acid was isolated in 1867 and in 1937 it was demonstrated that this substance cures the disease pellagra. The name niacin is derived from "nicotinic acid" and "vitamin".

Niacin is mainly involved in reactions that generate energy in tissues by the biochemical degradation of carbohydrates, fats and proteins. B3 functions in reductive biosynthesis such as the synthesis of fatty acids and cholesterol.

Benefits Of Niacin

Niacin improves blood circulation and helps prevent hypertension, atherosclerosis, abnormal blood clotting and stroke by lowering elevated fibrinogen levels. Niacin may prevent heart attacks and reduce the recurrence rate for second heart attacks by 30%; it may also alleviate Raynaud's disease by improving blood circulation to the hands and feet. B3 is useful for the treatment of age-related macular degeneration (ARMD).

Nicotinic acid may inhibit the ability of *candida glabrata* to cause urinary tract infections (by inhibiting the ability of *candida glabrata* to adhere to the epithelial cells of the urinary tract).

Niacin may reduce the mortality rate of cancer patients and may help to prevent some forms of cancer; B3 may decrease the rate of recurrence of bladder cancer in people treated with gamma-rays in radiation therapy, and may help prevent endometrial cancer.

Dietary Sources

Nicotinamide and nicotinic acid occur widely in nature. Nicotinic acid is more prevalent in plants and nicotinamide is more prevalent in animals. Yeast, liver, poultry, lean meats, nuts and legumes all contain niacin. Milk and green leafy vegetables provide lesser amounts. In cereal products, especially corn and wheat, nicotinic acid is bound to individual components and is not bioavailable. Specific food processing, such as the treatment of maize with lime water in the traditional preparation of tortillas in Mexico and Central America, increases the bioavailability of nicotinic acid.

Tryptophan contributes as much as two-thirds of the niacin activity required by adults in typical diets. Important food sources of tryptophan are meat, milk and eggs. There is no evidence that niacin from foods causes adverse effects.

Deficiency

Copper deficiency can inhibit the conversion of tryptophan to niacin. The drug penicillamine has been demonstrated to inhibit the tryptophan-to-niacin pathway in humans. This may be due in part to the copper chelating effect of penicillamine. The pathway from tryptophan to niacin is sensitive to a variety of nutritional alterations. Inadequate iron, riboflavin or vitamin B6 status reduces the synthesis of niacin from tryptophan. Other drugs which interact with niacin metabolism may also lead to niacin deficiency, e.g. tranquilizers (diazepam) and anticonvulsants (phenytoin, phenobarbital).

Moderate Deficiency Symptoms

- insomnia
- loss of appetite
- weight and strength loss
- soreness of the tongue and mouth
- indigestion
- abdominal pain
- burning sensations in various parts of the body
- vertigo
- headaches
- numbness
- nervousness
- poor concentration
- apprehension
- confusion and forgetfulness

Severe Deficiency

- pellagra, a disease characterized by dermatitis
- diarrhea and dementia
- in the skin, a pigmented rash develops symmetrically in areas exposed to sunlight (the term pellagra comes from the Italian phrase for raw skin)
- bright red tongue
- stomatitis (inflammation of the mucous tissue lining the mouth)
- vomiting and diarrhea
- headaches

- fatigue
- depression
- apathy
- loss of memory (neurological symptoms of pellagra)
- death (when untreated, pellagra is fatal)

Pharmacological doses of nicotinic acid, but not nicotinamide, exceeding 300 mg per day have been associated with a variety of side effects including nausea, diarrhea and transient flushing of the skin. Doses exceeding 2.5 gram per day have been associated with hepatotoxicity, glucose intolerance, hyperglycemia, elevated blood uric acid levels, heartburn, nausea and headaches. Severe jaundice may occur, even with doses as low as 750 mg per day, and may eventually lead to irreversible liver damage. Doses of 1.5 to 5 gram per day of nicotinic acid have been associated with blurred vision and other eye problems.

It is my opinion that niacin should be taken with or as part of a B-complex program, and at the recommended lower levels. As with all supplements, more is not better and they should be just one part of a healthy dietary lifestyle.

Vitamin D, More Than Sunshine

We often hear information about the merits of vitamin D. Along with this information comes an astounding amount of myth, misunderstanding and confusion.

In the 1920s and 1930s, a researcher and dentist by the name of Dr. Weston A. Price discovered what he called *Factor X*, which is found in dairy foods and fish oils. He found that butter made from spring milk was not only richer and darker in color, but also higher in nutrients. Dr. Price learned that individuals whose diets were high in Factor X were far less susceptible to cavities, tuberculosis and chronic health issues. Later, Factor X was renamed vitamin D and vitamin A. Physiologically each of us should be capable of producing upwards of 20,000 IU of vitamin D from fifteen to twenty minutes of sun exposure to the skin without sunscreen. Sadly, this is often not the case and research shows that the majority of the world's population is vitamin D deficient.

For many years physicians believed vitamin D was toxic when given in doses over 400 IU for prolonged periods. We now know that vitamin D is essential for bone health; but that is just the tip of the iceberg.

Research shows that vitamin D not only prevents bone loss, but according to John Jacob Cannell, MD, founder of the non-profit Vitamin D Council, "Current research indicates vitamin D deficiency plays a role in causing seventeen varieties of cancer as well as heart disease, stroke, hypertension, autoimmune diseases, diabetes, depression, chronic pain, osteoarthritis, osteoporosis, muscle weakness, muscle wasting, birth defects and periodontal disease."

Research shows there is a world of difference between synthetic vitamin D analogs, D2 and D3 (cholecalciferol). Toxicity occurs whenever we place a synthetic into our bodies. Natural forms of vitamin D3 (cholecalciferol) derived from lanolin are safe and effective at higher levels. The current RDA standards for vitamin D are pitifully low, at 200 to 600 IU. Healthy vitamin D blood levels are between 50-80 ng/ml, levels obtained by fewer than 5% of Americans.

The Vitamin D Council, one of the largest research bodies on vitamin D3, has found children through individuals in their 20s should be consuming 2000 IU of vitamin D3 daily—not vitamin D2, which is toxic to the liver. Adults 20 years and older should be consuming 5000+ IU daily for optimal health. The elderly, homebound or chronically ill are at greatest risk for vitamin D3 deficiency. Many individuals with blood levels of vitamin D3 lower than 32 ng/ml often respond best to injectable vitamin D3 therapy.

In 2006, Mary L. Hagood, MS, FNP-C and I began testing vitamin D levels in our clients. What we found in our small clinical study supported the information we had heard from the Vitamin D Council and from Ellie Campbell, DO, in North Carolina. The following is some of the information we gathered.

From 2006 to 2014 we saw 580 Caucasian men and women with an average age of 41; these individuals worked at various professions and those who worked outside had levels just as low as those who were elderly, homebound or living with chronic illness. Of these 580 clients, we had five participants who were within the optimum range on their 25-Hydroxy D3 test; they were all women over the age of 60 who had been supplementing with 5000 IU of vitamin D3 daily for over ten years.

Our sampling included 149 men and 431 women; of this total, 345 of the participants needed or were using bio-identical hormones for the thyroid and sex hormone replacement. Twenty-nine of the female participants had abnormal thermographic breast scans and were on an estrogen-free diet, using supplemental iodine and natural progesterone to lower breast cancer risk. Of these, 398 participants took part in injectable vitamin D3 supplementation administered monthly by Mary L. Hagood, MS, FNP-C. Dosage was 100,000 IU with 5000 IU taken orally daily.

When lab values were reviewed, we found our lowest 25-Hydroxy level was 5.0 in an 84-year-old male who had undergone a quadruple bypass eight years earlier and was a World War II veteran dependent on the VA hospital for his care. Next lowest level was 9.0 in a 47-year-old female of English ancestry who was a professional landscaper who worked outside an average of 300 days a year. Our next two lowest levels were 9.5; one was a male in his mid-fifties with brittle type 1 diabetes and the second was his wife and caregiver who suffered from severe depression and anxiety. These four individuals required additional vitamin D therapy at higher doses for an additional year after the eight months we recommended for the remainder of our client study base; their current levels are still lower than optimum.

A very active mother and wife had a level of 12. She is a third-generation Irish American with very fair skin, blue eyes and dark hair. She was teetering on the edge of metabolic syndrome and type 2 diabetes. Her vitamin D levels are still below the optimum range as she was unable to participate in the injectable vitamin D program; she is looking at potentially ten years of taking 5000 IU orally to reach the 32 mark on lab tests. By then she will be well into perimenopause or menopause and all the deficiency illness complications increase twofold by that time.

At the end of the study period, we were introduced to a lovely woman and mother of twins, who was morbidly obese weighing 426 pounds, and about to have gastric bypass surgery. Her lower spine was very painful, and the response from her primary care providers was to harrangue her about her weight and eating habits. Upon testing, her vitamin D3 levels were found to be 17. On average, this client consumed 1,000 calories daily, was active at home and worked. She had a family history of obesity and rickets.

The clients with the lowest values of vitamin D were all of northern European decent. All participants currently reside in Oregon, with 50 of the participants having relocated from other states within the last five years. In the 29 women with abnormal breast scans or breast cancer, vitamin D levels were found to be very low in addition to them having low levels of progesterone.

Blood tests were done on the study participants every four months to determine dosage; additionally, clients' calcium, potassium and magnesium levels were monitored. Vitamin K2 was added to the protocol for those receiving the injectable vitamin D to protect kidneys from excess calcium spilling.

Additionally, vitamin A was added to the protocol to improve the availability of the vitamin D to cell receptor sites.

By administering vitamin D3 shots clinicians are able to, in essence, fill the client's empty reserve and primary fuel tank of vitamin D without involving the kidneys and liver. Many clients will find a marked increase in energy and a reduction in pain and depression within 72 hours of their first shot. This therapy was done in a four-to eight-shot series based on the client's repeat 25-Hydroxy blood test at months four and eleven.

Northern European Ancestry

There is a correlation between individuals of northern European ancestry and low vitamin D levels. Many of these individuals are prone to digestive disorders such as IBS (Irritable Bowel Syndrome), ulcerative colitis (IBD), gluten sensitivity and thyroid problems. Possibly, the reason for this lies in the digestive system's inability to manufacture healthy levels of vitamin D. Clinical research supports the use of injectable vitamin D3 for individuals with low D3 blood levels. This is determined by the health practitioner requesting a 25-Hydroxy blood test.

For other individuals, oral or sublingual supplements may be adequate to restore healthy levels. The use of cod liver oil is not advised for those with low levels as it could prove potentially toxic due to high vitamin A at the doses necessary to reach optimal D3 blood levels. It is best to have your blood levels tested before beginning vitamin D therapies. This can be done through ZRT, Lab Corp or Life Extension Labs. There have been calibration issues with some of the other labs.

157,000 AMERICANS DIE FROM CORONARY ARTERY DISEASE EACH YEAR

A study published in June 2008 showed that men with low vitamin D levels suffer 2.42 times more heart attacks. Each year about 157,000 Americans die from coronary artery disease-related heart attacks. If every American optimized their vitamin D levels the numbers of deaths prevented would be 92,500. According to the latest study, men with higher vitamin D levels had a 142% reduction in heart attacks. The American Heart Association estimated that the annual cost of health care services, medications and lost productivity related to heart attacks is over 156 billion dollars. *(FoodBev.com | News | Coffee breaks are good for us. (n.d.). Retrieved from http://www.foodbev.com/news/coffee-breaks-are-good-for-us_br)*

At the American Heart Association's 49th Annual Conference on Cardiovascular Disease Epidemiology and Prevention, Jared P. Reis, PhD, and his team of researchers at Johns Hopkins Bloomberg School of Public Health, in Baltimore, announced their findings of a study of 3,577 adolescents, 12 to 19 years old (51 percent boys). "We showed strong associations between low levels of vitamin D and higher risk of high blood pressure, hyperglycemia and metabolic syndrome among adolescents, confirming the results of studies among adults," Dr. Reis said. Children and teenagers with the lowest levels of vitamin D were 2.36 times more likely to have hypertension, 2.54 times more likely to have high blood sugar and about 4 times more likely to have metabolic syndrome—a group of cardiovascular disease and diabetes risk factors that includes an increased waist circumference, high blood pressure, elevated triglycerides, low levels of high-density lipoprotein (HDL or "good") cholesterol and high fasting glucose levels.

There is a worldwide epidemic of vitamin D insufficiency, and the U.S. government is promoting illness management with high-cost pharmaceuticals instead of cost-effective nutritional supplements. Banning junk foods from schools and replacing vitamin D-robbing fluorescent lighting with skylights, LED or full spectrum lights could be a far better use of resources.

If every American achieved optimum vitamin D levels, a minimum savings of 84 billion dollars in health care costs could be realized. If we add up all the money saved by promoting wellness care through nutrition and lifestyle to the 84 billion, the U.S. would not have a healthcare crisis.

Currently, Medicare has discontinued vitamin D3 25-Hydroxy blood testing as a way of curbing escalating medical costs that are bankrupting the Medicare system. Wouldn't it be better to look at more cost-effective therapies, real wellness management and improved food quality, and reduce unnecessary and low efficacy medications? In Traditional Chinese Medicine you pay the doctor to keep you well; if you become ill, your care is free. I believe this model is one we could all benefit from.

It seems that every year we hear news reports that claim nutritional supplements are a waste of money— especially vitamin E. Major media companies appear to take delight in telling only part of the story, the part that looks the worst. The volume of information they don't tell you is the part that may save your life.

The term vitamin E covers eight fat-soluble compounds found in nature. Four of them are called tocopherols and the other four are called tocotrienols. In 2010, researchers found 8 additional forms, bringing the list up to 16. The name *tocopherols* derives from the Greek words *tocos*, meaning childbirth, and *pherein*, meaning to bring forth. The name was coined to highlight its essential role in the reproduction of various animal species. The ending -*ol* identifies the substance as being an alcohol.

The importance of vitamin E in humans was not accepted until relatively recently. Because its deficiency is not manifested by a well-recognized, widespread vitamin deficiency disease such as scurvy (vitamin C deficiency) or rickets (vitamin D deficiency), science has been late to recognize the importance of vitamin E.

Depletion of vitamin E tissue stores takes a very long time; no overt clinical deficiency symptoms have been noted in otherwise healthy adults. Symptoms of vitamin E deficiency are seen in patients with fat malabsorption syndromes or liver disease, in individuals with genetic defects affecting the α-tocopherol transfer protein and in newborn infants, particularly premature infants.

Vitamin E deficiency results in neuropathy, muscle weakness and pigmented retinopathy. Additionally, complications associated with type 2 diabetes, breast cancer, gluten sensitivity, Crohn's disease, ulcerative colitis, cirrhosis, high cholesterol, fatty liver and hepatitis result from vitamin E deficiency. Early diagnostic signs are leakage of muscle enzymes, increased plasma levels of lipid peroxidation products and increased red blood cells. In premature infants, vitamin E deficiency is associated with anemia, hemorrhage and fibroplasia.

A Little History

1922   Vitamin E is discovered by Evans and Scott Bishop

1936   Researchers isolate α-tocopherol in its pure form from wheat germ oil

1938   Nobel laureate Karrer synthesizes dl-α-tocopherol.

1945   The first antioxidant theory of vitamin E activity is proposed

1968   The Food and Nutrition Board of the U.S .National Research Council recognizes   vitamin E as an essential nutrient for humans

1977   Human vitamin E deficiency syndromes are described

1980   Vitamin E may prevent carcinogenic oxidative products of unsaturated fatty acids

1980s Vitamin E is demonstrated to be the major lipid-soluble antioxidant protecting cell membranes.

1990   Effectiveness of vitamin E in inhibiting LDL (low-density lipoprotein) oxidation is shown

2004   Vitamin E regulates gene expression in the liver and the testes of rats

Dietary Sources

Vegetable oils, nuts, whole grains and wheat germ are the main dietary sources of vitamin E. Other sources are seeds and green leafy vegetables. The vitamin E content of vegetables, fruits, dairy products, fish and meat is relatively low.

Vitamin E is absorbed together with lipids in the small intestine, depending on adequate pancreatic function and biliary secretion. Vitamin E is found in most human body tissues. The highest vitamin E contents are found in the adipose tissue, liver and muscles. The pool of vitamin E in the plasma, liver, kidneys and spleen turns over rapidly, whereas turnover of the content of adipose tissue is slow.

Vitamin E is thought to play a role in preventing heart disease and stroke due to its effects on a number of steps in the development of atherosclerosis (e.g. inhibition of LDL oxidation, inhibition of smooth muscle cell proliferation, inhibition of platelet adhesion, aggregation and platelet release reaction). Recent studies suggest vitamin E enhances immunity in the elderly, and that supplementation with vitamin E lowers the risk of contracting an upper respiratory tract infection, particularly the common cold.

Researchers are investigating the role of vitamin E in protecting against pollutants and lowering the risk of cancer and cataracts. Vitamin E in combination with vitamin C may protect the body from oxidative stress caused by extreme sports (e.g. ultra marathon running). Currently under investigation is the role of vitamin E supplementation in the treatment of Alzheimer's and ALS.

A large Northwestern Medicine® study done in 2014 ties the increasing consumption of supposedly healthy vitamin E-rich oils—canola, soybean and corn—to the rising incidence of lung inflammation and asthma.

> *"The new study shows drastically different health effects of vitamin E depending on its form. The form of Vitamin E called gamma-tocopherol in the ubiquitous soybean, corn and canola oils is associated with decreased lung function in humans, the study reports. The other form of Vitamin E, alpha-tocopherol, which is found in olive and sunflower oils, does the opposite. It is associated with better lung function.*
>
> *"Considering the rate of affected people we found in this study, there could be 4.5 million individuals in the U.S. with reduced lung function as a result of their high gamma-tocopherol consumption," said senior author Joan Cook-Mills, an associate professor of medicine in allergy/immunology at Northwestern University Feinberg School of Medicine.*
>
> *This is the first study to show gamma-tocopherol is associated with worse lung function."* [160]

When selecting a vitamin E supplement, be sure to buy a complete blend of alpha, beta, delta and gamma tocopherols. They should be extracted from natural sources and come from a highly reputable company. Adding vitamin E to a wholesome natural diet will help you to take control of your health.

---

[160] Northwestern University. "Vitamin E in canola, other oils hurts lungs." ScienceDaily. ScienceDaily, 20 May 2014. <www.sciencedaily.com/releases/2014/05/140520220424.htm>.

Vitamin K is a fat-soluble vitamin. It has received far less attention from the media and public than its more famous "cousins" A, D and E. Vitamin K occurs naturally in two forms: vitamin K1, found in plants; vitamin K2, which is synthesized by bacteria in the intestinal tract of humans and various animals. Vitamin K3 is a synthetic compound and it is only used in animal nutrition.

Research over the last 25 years has given a new and expanded view of vitamin K. It is now known to be essential to bone and brain health, and to help prevent atherosclerosis and calcified arterial plaque.

A Little History

In Denmark in 1929, Henrik Dam observed that chicks fed on fat-free diets developed hemorrhages and started bleeding. He subsequently proposed that the antihemorrhagic substance was a new fat-soluble vitamin, which he called vitamin K (after the first letter of the Danish word "Koagulation"). In 1939, Vitamin K1 was synthesized by Doisy and associates.

What Vitamin K2 Can Do

Vitamin K2 protects against excess bone resorption by turning off excess osteoclast activity, and it supports the critical role of new bone formation by enabling osteocalcin to pull calcium from the blood and layer it onto the bone. Vitamin K2 has proven to be as effective as prescription drugs in reducing the incidence of bone fractures.

A Japanese study in postmenopausal women compared the effect of K2 with the drug Didronel® on the incidence of vertebral (spine) fracture. Women taking K2 at a dose of 45 mg per day experienced a fracture rate of 8.0% compared with 8.7% for those taking the drug therapy. Furthermore, women taking both K2 and the drug experienced only a 3.8% fracture rate. In a placebo group that received neither K2 nor drug therapy, nearly 21% of women experienced bone fractures.

The Nurses' Health Study followed 72,000 women for 10 years and found women whose vitamin K intakes were in the lowest quintile (1/5) had a 30% higher risk of hip fracture than women with vitamin K intakes in the highest four quintiles.

The Framingham Heart Study, a seven-year study in over 888 elderly men and women, found men and women with dietary vitamin K intakes in the highest quartile (1/4) had a 65% lower risk of hip fracture than those with dietary vitamin K intakes in the lowest quartile (approximately 254 mcg vs. 56 mcg of vitamin K).

Vitamin K shows promise in the prevention and treatment of numerous cancers, including prostate cancer.

Individuals who take Coumadin® have long been advised to avoid vitamin K; as a result, they may suffer increased atherosclerosis and osteoporosis. Under a doctor's supervision, vitamin K can help stabilize blood indicators of coagulation in Coumadin® users while conferring other health benefits.

By preventing pathological tissue calcification, vitamin K may confer anti-aging effects throughout the body.

Higher vitamin K intake has been associated with reduced all-cause mortality.

Vitamin K2 & Heart Health

In 2004, a ground-breaking seven-year study of 4,800 subjects (the Rotterdam Study) linked K2 intake with a reduced risk of coronary heart disease (CHD). Researchers found those with higher levels of vitamin K2 in their diets experienced lower death rates from heart disease and less deposition of calcium in the aorta compared with subjects with minimal K2 intake. K1 did not confer this benefit. The researchers concluded, "Our findings suggest a protective effect of K2 intake against CHD, which could be mediated by inhibition of arterial calcification. ... Adequate intake of K2 may contribute to CHD prevention."

In a current study, researchers set out to compare the effects of vitamin K1 and K2 on arterial health. The results indicated that 62% (360) of the women had coronary calcification. Subjects with the highest vitamin K2 intakes experienced a 20% reduction in calcification of the arteries. According to the researchers, "This study shows high dietary vitamin K2 intake is associated with reduced coronary calcification. Adequate vitamin K2 intakes could therefore be important in the prevention of cardiovascular disease."

Vitamin K2 plays a vital role in ensuring that calcium stays in the bones—maintaining adequate bone mineral density—and out of the arteries. It is an essential cofactor for a chemical process known as carboxylation, which enables calcium-regulating proteins to perform their functions.

In Febuary of 2015 a landmark study was released in *Thrombosis and Haemostasis, the International Journal for Vascular Biology and Medicine*. It was the first study "showing the beneficial effect of long-term vitamin K2 (menaquinone-7 or MK-7) use on cardiovascular health. The randomized, double-blind, placebo-controlled clinical trial using a specific vitamin K2 called MenaQ7, made by NattoPharma, proved the supplement's positive cardiovascular effects by improving arterial flexibility."[161]

Dietary Sources

The best dietary sources of vitamin K1 are green leafy vegetables such as spinach, broccoli, Brussels sprouts, cabbage and lettuce. Other rich sources are certain vegetable oils. Good sources include oats, potatoes, tomatoes, asparagus and butter. Lower levels are found in beef, pork, ham, organ meats, egg yolks, fermented dairy products, the Japanese fermented soybean dish, natto, milk, carrots, corn, most fruits and many other vegetables. High-quality K2 supplements are recommended for anyone wanting to prevent CHD or osteoporosis.

---

[161] www.reuters.com/article/2015/02/19/idUSnMKW7j9M2a+1c4+MKW20150219

Every year, millions of women in their thirties and forties are given sleep aids, antidepressants and anti-anxiety medications. They sign up for gym memberships and go on calorie-restrictive or fad diets to lose or maintain weight. For years we have known about the health challenges facing women going through menopause but little is discussed about the years before "the change".

Menopause can be a difficult time for women. Our society does not tend to see the changes in hormones and body structure as a freeing or an arousing time in a woman's life. For some, the years before menopause (perimenopause) may be wrought with indecision, stress, frustration, weight gain, wrinkles and fear. Our ability to cope with stress, our self-esteem and our libido may not be what it once was.

Wine and chocolate often become the drugs of choice during this time frame. Eating habits have a profound impact on how easy or hard the lifestyle and hormone transitions may turn out to be. Men also have aging challenges, and the foods they eat will determine their vitality, muscle mass, weight, sex drive, cognition, mental health, and heart disease and diabetes risk factors.

Ladies First

So what is peri-menopause? This is the time in a woman's reproductive years when her hormones begin "stuttering". Changing hormone levels, particularly estrogens and progesterone, cause perimenopausal symptoms that continue for a year or two after menopause. As ovulation becomes more erratic, the intervals between menstration may be longer or shorter, menstrual flow may be scanty to profuse, and some periods may be missed. Some women have mild perimenopausal symptoms. Others have severe symptoms that affect their sleep and daily lives.

Changes in sexual function. During perimenopause, sexual arousal may change. Most women who had satisfactory sexual intimacy before perimenopause will continue to do so; some report that *better* is the word for this time in a woman's sexual life.

When estrogens (the female body makes five estrogens) levels diminish, your vaginal tissues may lose lubrication and elasticity, making intercourse painful. Low estrogen, progesterone and testosterone levels may also leave you more vulnerable to urinary or vaginal infections. Vaginal itching or dryness, causing discomfort during sexual activity, can be related to low testosterone levels as well as low progesterone. The human body has hormone receptors everywhere and these hormones are heavily utilized by muscles, organs and the brain. In fact, there are more hormone receptors in the brain than throughout the rest of the body, which accounts for why hormone shifts have such a profound effect on thought patterns and brain chemistry.

Mood changes. Some women experience mood swings, headaches, foggy brain, short term memory loss, increased frustration, anger, irritability or depression during perimenopause; the cause of these symptoms may be sleep disruption and hormone shifts.

Sleep problems and hot flashes. Sleep problems are common; you may feel exhausted but just can't seem to stop your mind from racing, or night sweats may wake you. About 65 to 75 percent of women experience hot flashes during perimenopause. Their intensity, duration and frequency vary.

Weight gain and loss of bone. Weight gain is common as estrogens become dominant in the body, replacing hormones like progesterone and testosterone. When the balance of hormones is disrupted, insulin resistance increases, raising the risks for type 2 diabetes and heart disease. Bone loss may increase during this time if a woman is not proactive about weight-lifting exercise and the right forms of mineral supplementation.

Heart palpitations may be noticed for the first time; this is associated with declining progesterone levels. Progesterone IVs are used in emergency rooms for women with tachycardia complaints.

Cholesterol and blood pressure levels may rise, indicating metabolic syndrome. Declining hormone levels may lead to unfavorable changes in cholesterol levels, including an increase in low-density lipoprotein (LDL) cholesterol. At the same time, high-density lipoprotein (HDL) cholesterol decreases in many women. Additionally, blood pressure may begin increasing; this is due in part to the decline in progesterone which has a natural thinning effect on blood and is involved in regulating water retention.

Vaginal and bladder problems make an appearance. Loss of tissue tone may contribute to urinary incontinence. HRT (synthetic hormone replacement; eg. Premarin™) therapies are known to increase urinary incontinence issues.

Salivary hormone testing allows health care providers to clearly see which hormones are low and to efficiently help the client manage their hormone levels. With the right information and proactive healthcare providers working in partnership with you, these years can be more rewarding. Look for a qualified bio-identical hormone practitioner in your area or contact ZRT laboratory for information.

Fat Facts for Women

I freely admit I am over forty, female and fighting to keep my weight under control; no matter how good we are, we still can gain weight on water. What is with that?

If you were born between 1944 and 1959, you belong to the generation that came of age when the diet industry developed. You were first told to clean your plate and be mindful of starving children. Later you were told that the ideal figure was delicate and Twiggy-esque. This preceded a wave of "crash diets". The curvy Marilyn Monroe bombshells of the 1940s and 50s were no longer *en vogue*.

The Greek word *diata* denoted a healthy lifestyle. The English translation came to mean not only the manner in which we eat but what we consume. Modern connotations suggest our daily fare should be subject to limitation in order to lose weight—*to die with a t*. Women over forty have been sent the message for decades now that there is something wrong with their appearance and that there is a quick fix available in a spray, bottle or pill.

In the 1960s, "diet doctors" were medical practitioners who utilized therapies such as diet pills. In the 1970s, 8% of all prescriptions written in the U.S. were for amphetamines, 2 billion of them specifically prescribed for weight loss. By 1999 the sales of commercial diet programs, foods, books, appetite suppressants, hospital weight loss programs, health clubs, surgeries and spas reached more than $30 billion a year. On any given day at least 20% of the population is dieting.

In 1997 the CDC announced that for the first time in history, there were more overweight and obese adults than the average-sized adult and that 1 out of 4 children were overweight. Physical fitness levels had plummeted in adults and children; children were being excused from PE classes because they were unable to handle the standard activity levels.

Diets fail because no one can stay on them for prolonged periods. During times of stress the human brain looks for ways to balance chemistry; food is used to self-medicate. Busy and stressed, we reach for convenient foods instead of fresh and healthy ones; burnt out and drained, we wind up on the couch instead of out walking laps.

"After the age of forty the rules of self-care for women change. You can no longer look to fad diets, or continue to eat the same as when we were in our twenties. In fact, if you continue to eat the same amount of calories as you did when twenty until the age of forty-five, you can expect to gain at least thirty to fifty pounds and the increasing health challenges that go along with perimenopause and weight gain if you don't make proactive changes," says Dr. Pamela Peeke, MD.[162]

A study by the National Institutes of Health, released in 2000, concluded that women whose waists measure thirty-five inches or greater are at risk of disease and early death. Women in their perimenopausal years, the last major hormonal transition of life, can experience a sort of "shape-shifting". The average weight gain during the 7-10 years surrounding the onset of menopause can range from 10 to 25 pounds. Instead of accumulating around the hips and thighs, the weight settles around the waist. Women's metabolisms traditionally decline at a rate of 5% per decade of life, starting at age twenty. At twenty you may need roughly 2,000 to 2,500 calories per day (one fast food take-out meal or two slices of pizza exceeds this amount) to live. By the time you are forty-five, you could require about 300 calories less per day. If you continue to consume the extra calories, you will gain 1 pound every twelve days, or 30 pounds per year.

---

[162] (Pamela Peeke, 2000)

A slowing metabolism, loss of muscle mass and unhealthy lifestyle can compound the natural changes of the menopausal years. Chronic stress never allows the body to shut down and rejuvenate. It is paramount for women to learn to care for themselves and to find ways to unload the tension, anxiety and fatigue associated with stress.[163] A regular yoga workout, daily walk, gardening or spiritual practices can help mitigate the stress that slows the female metabolism.

Women who expose their bodies to toxic stress and prolonged periods of elevated cortisol activate the "refueling response", potentially resulting in bouts of binge eating or mindless eating. The stressed-out eater may then turn to fad diets to lose weight, which creates even more stress, resulting in food deprivation. Current research has found that if stress goes on long enough, bodies cannot return to homeostasis and health begins to break down. It is now known that the most common diseases are largely due to a malfunctioning of the adaptive response to stress, rather than the direct damage done by germs.[164]

Estrogens tend to hold fluid in the body while progesterone has a mild diuretic action. Estrogens are powerful activators of fat storage in the hips, thighs and buttocks.[165, 166] During perimenopause, estrogen and progesterone levels become more erratic and the storage site for fat shifts to the waistline. All the sex hormones begin to decline, except for testosterone (in some individuals), which can increase and stimulate the creation of more abdominal fat. Insulin, another powerful hormone, also acts to increase fat storage and exacerbate inflammation, leading to heart disease and diabetes. Fluctuations in women's weight happen monthly, naturally: "It's well known that women undergo hormonal changes every month due to the menstrual cycle. These changes can cause women to eat more, which is a natural, biological occurrence." Said, Kelly Klump Michigan State University Foundation Professor

Professor, Kelly Klump, has found the increased food intake causes some women to become much more preoccupied with their body weight and shape. Women are biologically wired to increase their food intake during their monthly cycle in preparation for pregnancy.

Klump says that the changes in food intake are all part of a natural, evolutionary process. "In our culture, we tend to view any increased eating by a woman as a negative thing, even when it is biologically and evolutionarily driven," Klump said.

---

[163] (Robert E. Thayer, 2001)
[164] (Shawn Talbott, 2007)
[165] (Kenna Stephenson, 2004)
[166] (Pamela Wartian Smith, HRT: The Answers, 2003)

"This is a potentially dangerous chain of events that could lead to severe and life-threatening eating disorders, including anorexia nervosa and bulimia nervosa."[167]

Lean mass is one of the strongest determinants of bone mass throughout life. Until now, it has been unclear whether fat mass and lean mass differ in how they influence bone development in boys and girls. Findings from previous studies have been inconsistent regarding whether fat mass has a positive or negative impact on bone development. This new study shows that fat mass is a strong stimulus for the accrual of cortical bone mass (hard outer layer of bone) in girls.[168]

When you lose weight, where does the fat go? Most of the mass is expelled as carbon dioxide. A study published in 2014 stated that: "Despite a worldwide obsession with diets and fitness regimes, many health professionals cannot correctly answer the question of where body fat goes when people lose weight. The most common misconception among doctors, dieticians and personal trainers is the missing mass has been converted into energy or heat. The correct answer is that most of the mass is breathed out as carbon dioxide and goes into thin air."[169]

For every pound of muscle mass lost due to crash diets (8 lbs after the first diet and 16 lbs after the second) a woman has decreased her metabolic rate by 35 to 50 calories. This means that if she doesn't consume 500-800 fewer calories per day she will gain back all the weight she lost plus more. It makes much more sense to build muscle, which increases your metabolic rate so you can eat healthy foods in reasonable amounts. This also lowers stress and keeps weight under control.[170]

The "non-diet approach" to weight management is more useful in worksite wellness programs, a 2014 study reported. "The vast majority of wellness programs limit their approach to promoting diets, which may result in participants regaining the majority of their weight once the programs end. Now, researchers at the University of Missouri have found 'Eat for Life', a new wellness approach that focuses on mindfulness and intuitive eating as a lifestyle, is more effective than traditional weight-loss programs in improving individuals' views of their bodies and decreasing

---

[167] Michigan State University. "Fluctuations in women's weight happens monthly, naturally." ScienceDaily. ScienceDaily, 16 December 2014. <www.sciencedaily.com/releases/2014/12/141216123821.htm>.
[168] The Endocrine Society. "Fat mass helps build bone mass in girls, study suggests; excessive fat reduction may increase osteoporosis risk." ScienceDaily. ScienceDaily, 7 January 2010. <www.sciencedaily.com/releases/2010/01/100105095844.htm>.
[169] University of New South Wales. "When you lose weight, where does the fat go? Most of the mass is breathed out as carbon dioxide, study shows." ScienceDaily. ScienceDaily, 16 December 2014. <www.sciencedaily.com/releases/2014/12/141216212047.htm>.
[170] (Pamela Wartian Smith, Demystifying Weight Loss, 2007)

problematic eating behaviors."[171] This holistic approach takes stress out of the equation.

The younger a woman is when she goes on her first diet, the more likely she is to experience several adverse health outcomes later in life.[172] The fad diet trend needs to be replaced with a naturally balanced and healthy lifestyle.

Cortisol may be responsible for weight gain as well as fatigue. It is also implicated in diabetes, fibromyalgia, heart disease, poor immune function and more. In 2014, the United Kingdom listed obesity as an illness. To what extent is stress the root cause of this "illness"?

Mammograms: A Different Perspective

Millions of women regularly schedule mammograms to monitor their breast health. A surprising number are terrified of the potential for developing breast cancer; this is partly due to well-intentioned media coverage sponsored by medical groups. My own insurance company began mailing me reminders to have a mammogram when I turned fifty.

My response then was the same as it is today: No, thank you. I'm not a big fan of preventive testing; I find the terminology misleading at best and fraudulent at worst. In my opinion, there is no testing that is preventive; it should be more aptly thought of as "early detection". The only true prevention is a healthy lifestyle.

Breast cancer is on the rise and cause for concern, but repeatedly exposing delicate tissues to radiation is not necessary for monitoring purposes. The most common form of breast cancer, ductal carcinoma, is slow-growing and develops over ten to twelve years before it may be detected on a mammogram, according to many researchers. Other breast health monitoring options are available, without the risks that have been underplayed by radiologists. The radiologists, by the way, have their techs scurry into lead-shielded rooms before hitting the power button.

---

[171] University of Missouri-Columbia. "Non-diet approach to weight management more effective in worksite wellness programs." ScienceDaily. ScienceDaily, 7 July 2014.
<www.sciencedaily.com/releases/2014/07/140707134331.htm>.
[172] Society for the Study of Ingestive Behavior. "Dieting young may lead to poor health outcomes later: Trends in dieting strategies in young adult women from 1982 to 2012." ScienceDaily. ScienceDaily, 29 July 2014.
<www.sciencedaily.com/releases/2014/07/140729224908.htm>.

However, will your doctor or insurance company recognize the validity of other forms of breast health screening, such as thermographic imaging? Will they be willing to learn "new" technology (that has been utilized by the military for over 35 years)? Many of my clients have chosen to take matters into their own hands and have incorporated Thermographic Imaging of the Breast[173, 174, 175,] into their integrative health programs.

Note that I did not say thermographic imaging is an alternative to the mammogram, because it is not an alternative, according to the FDA or resistant medical establishments. That may change after a recent comprehensive review of mammograms .

On April 1, 2014, Harvard Medical School released a comprehensive review of fifty years of international studies assessing the potential benefits and harms of mammograms.

The summary states: "A comprehensive review of 50 years' worth of international studies assessing the benefits and harms of mammography screening suggests that the advantages of the screening are often overestimated, while harms are underestimated. The authors report that the best estimate of the reduction in mortality from breast cancer due to annual screening for women overall is about 19 percent. For women in their 40s, the reduction in risk was about 15 percent, and for women in their 60s, about 32 percent. But how much a woman benefits depends on her underlying risk of breast cancer.

"The researchers estimated that among 10,000 women in their 40s who undergo annual mammography for 10 years, about 190 will be diagnosed with breast cancer. Of those 190, the researchers estimate that about 5 will avoid death from breast cancer due to screening. About 25 of the 190 would die of breast cancer regardless of whether they have a mammogram or not."

In 2009, a study presented at the Radiological Society of North America reported: "Low-dose radiation from annual mammography screening may increase breast cancer risk in women with genetic or familial predisposition to breast cancer." In 2010, the Society of Breast Imaging and the American College of Radiology announced that women should begin annual mammograms at forty; earlier for high-risk patients. Later that same year, the headlines read:

---

[173] http://advancedthermography.com/Breast_Thermography_Image.php
[174] http://www.breastthermography.com/find-a-center.htm
[175] http://www.drrind.com/therapies/breast-thermography

"Radiation Fears Should Not Deter Women from Mammography Screening, Study Suggests." It seemed to me that the media blitz was more about saving market shares than saving women's health. *(Radiation fears should not deter women from mammography screening. (n.d.). Retrieved from http://phys.org/news/2010-11-deter-women-mammography-screening.html_br)*

Breast Health

For over five years, I hosted a guest practitioner who specialized in breast health, in addition to my direct medical oversight. The practitioners' findings on their first two visits to my office had me alarmed—out of the dozen women seen, six clients were found to have potential problems; three of them ended up having surgeries. One of the three had had a negative mammogram and ultrasound prior to her thermographic breast imaging. This compelled me to learn more about the biochemistry of breast cancer.

Breasts are mammary glands that are comprised of fat, tissues, muscles, lymph nodes and blood vessels. All of these components are affected by hormones, both naturally occuring and—like xenobiotic estrogens—introduced via food and the environment.

I first learned about the effects of xenobiotic toxins when I was on the Hepatitis C Task Force for Douglas County, Oregon. Vietnam veterans have a very high prevalence of Hepatitis C; many were exposed to Agent Orange which has now been linked with diabetes, endocrine disorders and heart disease. Herbicides, pesticides, fungicides, petroleum distillates and many other chemicals are transformed by the human body into xenobiotic estrogens that disrupt normal chemical pathways, leading to endocrine disruption and increased harmful estrogens that affect the heart, breast and prostate and can lead to diabetes.[176]

These chemical agents are liberally applied to roadways and used in landscaping, agriculture and construction. Petroleum products, including plastics, are detected along with prescription medications, pesticides and herbicides in city and rural water supplies. These contaminants increase cancer risk factors and are linked with increases in mood disorders, theoretically because of the xenobiotic interference with neurotransmitter pathways of the brain. Much of this I learned through David Zava, PhD, and his team at ZRT Lab in Beaverton, Oregon.

---

[176] ZRTLAB.com

The younger a woman is when she begins producing estrogens (or goes on synthetics) and the longer she is exposed to them, the greater her risk of developing heart disease[177] or breast cancer. There are several pharmaceuticals that remain in the human body for generations, being passed from mother to daughter's eggs in the womb. Could this be a causative factor in the most aggressive forms of cancer? The women who came of age from 1944 to 1969 were the first to use birth control pills and to be exposed to high levels of environmental estrogens. This age group is now seeing marked increases in "hot" breast scans, indicating high estrogen-driven inflammation.

As a woman enters perimenopause and later, menopause, her body stops producing essential hormones that keep estrogens in balance. She may become estrogen-dominant, her hormone receptor sites effectively smothered in estrogens. When estrogens are out of balance, heart disease, diabetes and cancer risks increase. Dr. Kenna Stephenson, MD, has shown in her landmark bio-identical studies that when women are returned to normal hormonal physiological ranges, diabetes, high cholesterol, depression, high blood pressure and menopausal symptoms all normalize. This is not the case with synthetic hormone replacement therapies, which can be detrimental.

The human body produces several forms of estrogen that are made from cholesterol: estradiol, estrone and estriol. They are needed by both women and men and are central to brain function, as are all the hormones. Estrogens are utilized in bones and muscle tissue. There are hormone receptor sites all over the body, with some of the highest concentrations in the brain.

The plant kingdom provides what are called phytoestrogens. Mexican wild yam, black cohosh, red clover, licorice, sage, unicorn root, soybean, flax seeds, hops and sesame seeds are a few examples of phytoestrogen-containing herbs and foods. For centuries, such plants have helped women maintain hormonal health. Now, with synthetic hormones and chemicals pervasive in our food, water, environment and prescription medications, we are seeing breast cancer climb to the second most prevalent form of cancer for women while prostate cancer is on the rise in men. Note also that heart-related illnesses are responsible for 52% of women's deaths in the United States; the heart is greatly affected by estrogen dominance.

---

[177] American Heart Association. "Women's age at first menstrual cycle linked to heart disease risk." ScienceDaily. ScienceDaily, 15 December 2014.
<www.sciencedaily.com/releases/2014/12/141215185203.htm>.

There is no easy fix for breast cancer, but with a combination of "early detection" testing, including thermographic imaging; dietary/detox and nutraceutical therapies; and proactively eliminating xenoestrogens and synthetic estrogens from your environment, risk factors can be reduced and potential problems can be averted before cancer forms.

Prevention & Detection

In the fall of 2009, the federal government announced it was changing the guidelines for when and how often women should have mammograms. For weeks I heard from concerned clients who felt that their only hope for breast cancer prevention was being taken away from them. This provided an opportunity to discuss their options, and to remind them that mammograms are on average 40% successful in finding cancer; they are a tool to help with early detection and not a method of prevention.

For millions of individuals with fibrocystic breast tissue, they can not only be painful but can cause inconclusive or false positive results. The anxiety, fear, stress and pain these individuals go through does little to prevent cancer and can actually increase risk factors. Ultrasound scanning helps increase the find rate of breast cancer, and when these two detection tools are combined with thermographic camera technology, cancers can be found while still very small or even before cancer cells have had a chance to metastasize and when delicate tissues are still in the inflammatory process. Thermographic cameras were first developed by the military and are actively used for battlefield triage; they are ideal for locating, without radiation or compression, areas of intense heat and inflammation (i.e., signs of potential cancer).

That breast density helps better predict breast cancer risk was a hot topic at the 2014 Breast Cancer Symposium in San Antonio, Texas. The study "Volumetric Breast Density Improves Breast Cancer Risk Prediction" was presented by Jennifer Harvey, MD, professor of radiology at the UVA School of Medicine. "Our current ability to accurately predict an individual woman's risk of developing breast cancer is very limited, which is why we mostly recommend the same screening for everyone," said Harvey. "The results of this study show that breast density significantly improves the accuracy of the breast cancer risk model, which is critical if screening recommendations are to be individualized.

The automated measurement of breast density proved to be one of the top five predictors of breast cancer risk in the study population."[178,179]

Prevention begins long before cancer forms, and for individuals who have undergone surgery and cancer treatment it is a must, if the increased odds of developing secondary cancers are to be reduced. The following recommendations are on the top of the list, in current cancer research, after expensive drugs.

Organic/ Sustainable Foods: One of the first areas to start is the kitchen. If it comes in a bag, box, can or jar, odds are good that it contains undesirable chemicals. Many food additives, fats and flavorings inhibit the body's ability to repair itself and protect against cancer. Fresh foods contain the key nutrients the immune system needs; they are also less likely to be contaminated with xenoestrogens from plastics and pesticides.[180]

On a related note, in the winter of 2014 I was stunned when the Susan G. Komen® Foundation came out in opposition to organic foods. This is a direct contradiction to many medical organizations' and practitioners' recommendations.

Iodine: Deficiency of dietary iodine causes a spectrum of disorders and is heavily implicated in breast cancer. A common misconception is that iodine's sole function is to act as an essential component of thyroid hormones. Accumulating evidence suggests that iodine has many benefits, including maintaining the integrity of the mammary gland, antioxidant functions, anti-tumor activities, detoxification, immune system strengthening and protection against potentially pathogenic bacteria. Iodine has been shown to induce death (apoptosis) in breast and thyroid cancer cells. Iodine helps the body to detoxify harmful chemicals that disrupt normal hormone function. [181] Please, make sure you test your iodine levels through reputable labs prior to adding this to your diet.

[178] University of Virginia Health System. "Breast density helps better predict breast cancer risk." ScienceDaily. ScienceDaily, 16 December 2014. <www.sciencedaily.com/releases/2014/12/141216100431.htm>.
[179] American Institute of Physics. "Diagnostic screening: Microwave imaging of the breast may be better and safer." ScienceDaily. ScienceDaily, 16 December 2014. <www.sciencedaily.com/releases/2014/12/141216113015.htm>.
[180] (Maureen Keane, 1996)
[181] (David Brownstein, Iodine - Why You Need It, 2006)

Vitamin D3: Women who have mutations in their vitamin D receptor gene are nearly twice as likely to develop breast cancer compared to women who do not have the mutation. The vitamin D receptor gene controls the action of vitamin D in the body. Scientists have found that Caucasian women with certain versions of this gene not only have an increased risk of breast cancer but also may suffer from a more aggressive form of the disease if it spreads. Different versions of the vitamin D receptor gene will influence the way vitamin D protects the female body against cancers.

Five to ten percent of breast cancer cases are due to already established gene mutations such as BRCA1. However, the underlying cause of breast cancer in women who do not have this gene and have no family history of the disease has remained a mystery. The mutation in the vitamin D receptor gene may have a role to play in disease development in women who would not ordinarily be expected to develop the disease. Fish, liver and egg yolk are the only foods that naturally contain vitamin D.

Proteolytic Enzymes: New York City immunologist Nicholas Gonzalez, MD, uses nutrients, enzymes and organic foods to treat cancer. Dr. Gonzalez was introduced to the cancer treatments of William Donald Kelley, DDS, and John Beard (1900) as a student. Kelley pioneered a successful method of using enzymes and nutrition for cancer treatment, and Scottish biologist Beard proposed that the digestive function and pancreatic enzymes represent the body's main defense against cancer. Enzymes are the cornerstone of health. Our trace minerals are the foundation where enzymes are the transport vehicles needed for utilization of nutrients by every cell. Enzymes are involved in every metabolic function in the body. Enzymes also play an essential role in inflammation regulation and immune system function. Proteolytic enzymes such as bromelain, papain, pancreatin, trypsin, chymotrypsin, serrapeptase and rutin are essential regulators and modulators of the inflammatory response. When immune complexes occur in excess, cancer and a host of other chronic illnesses are found to increase. Although individual proteolytic enzymes are useful, the extraordinary combination of enzymes yields a combination greater than its sum.

Buckwheat: Buckwheat is rich in phytochemicals including rutin, isoquercitrin, quercetin, catechin, myricetin and various anthocyanins. Buckwheat is also a dietary source of vitamin E, vitamin B6, zinc, copper, selenium and manganese. Components of buckwheat have been found to have antioxidant, anticarcinogenic, antimutagenic and antifungal properties. An extract of buckwheat hulls has been shown to have cytotoxic effects in human breast, liver and stomach cancer cells. A peptide of buckwheat seeds has been found to inhibit proliferation of liver and breast cancer cells, as well as leukemia cells. Tartary buckwheat (similar to buckwheat) has been found to have antiproliferative effects in human breast cancer cells. Buckwheat also has been shown to inhibit carcinogen-induced mammary tumors in laboratory rats by lowering circulating estrogen.[182, 183, 184]

Dr. James L. Wilson, who has introduced millions to the dangers of adrenal insufficiency through his presentations, book and website, explains the connection between cortisol and adrenal fatigue.

What Is Adrenal Fatigue?

According to James L. Wilson, ND, DC, PhD: "Adrenal fatigue is a collection of signs and symptoms, known as a 'syndrome', that results when the adrenal glands function below the necessary level. Most commonly associated with intense or prolonged stress, it can also arise during or after acute or chronic infections, especially respiratory infections such as influenza, bronchitis or pneumonia. As the name suggests, its paramount symptom is fatigue that is not relieved by sleep but it is not a readily identifiable entity like measles or a growth on the end of your finger. You may look and act relatively normal with adrenal fatigue and may not have any obvious signs of physical illness, yet you live with a general sense of unwellness, tiredness or 'gray' feelings. People suffering from adrenal fatigue often have to use coffee, colas and other stimulants to get going in the morning and to prop themselves up during the day."[185]

Our adrenal glands help us to deal with the varying forms of stress by manufacturing cortisol and a host of other hormones. In essence the adrenal glands are the backup generator for the hormones used by our cells. When menopause or andropause (male menopause) begin, the adrenal glands take over the production of some hormones like progesterone and testosterone. The more burden on the glands the more likely you are to develop midline weight gain, blood sugar imbalances, poor immune function and fatigue.

In today's world we are no longer being chased by lions and bears; our stressors are man-made, environmental and internal. Chronic illness is one stressor to look at; not

---

[182] http://foodforbreastcancer.com/foods/buckwheat

[183] http://www.ncbi.nlm.nih.gov/pubmed/21138372

[184] http://ftp.greenmedinfo.com/article/protease-inhibitors-buckwheat-seeds-are-active-against-human-t-acute-lymphoblastic-leukemia

[185] (James L. Wilson, 2007)

only is the person with the illness overworking their entire endocrine system but those who care for and love that person are overloading their adrenal glands as well. Studies have shown that those who fill caregiving roles have the highest levels of adrenal fatigue and the majority of them are women; working moms, teachers, nurses and home healthcare providers. [186]

Adrenal insufficiency or fatigue involves overworked, damaged or depleted adrenal glands. Addison's disease is a syndrome specifically related to inadequate secretion of corticosteroid hormones. Adrenal fatigue may be an underlying cause of hypotension (low blood pressure), alopecia areata ("patchy" hair loss) and suppression of the immune system, and one of the causes of chronic fatigue syndrome (CFS). The adrenal glands of CFS patients are, on average, only half of the size of normal, healthy persons. Adrenal insufficiency may cause fatigue and be an underlying cause of hypoglycemia (low blood sugar), impaired liver function, salt craving, anxiety, depression, poor concentration, excessive drowsiness, insomnia and memory impairment. [187]

What Does Cortisol Do?

Cortisol has diverse and highly important effects on regulating the metabolism of glucose, protein and fatty acids. Cortisol plays a role in mood and well-being, immune cells and inflammation, blood vessels and blood pressure and in the maintenance of connective tissue such as bones, muscle and skin. Under stressful conditions, cortisol generally maintains blood pressure and limits excess inflammation. Unfortunately, adrenal stress response can react by secreting too much cortisol.

Who Is Most Likely To Have Adrenal Fatigue?

Anyone can suffer from adrenal fatigue. An illness, life crisis or ongoing difficult situation can drain the adrenal resources of even the healthiest person. There are factors that can make you more prone to adrenal fatigue. These include lifestyle (poor diet, substance abuse, too little sleep, too many pressures); a chronic illness or repeated infections such as bronchitis or pneumonia; or having a mother who suffered from adrenal fatigue around the time of your birth. According to Dr. Wilson,

---

[186] (William McK. Jefferies, 1996)
[187] (James L. Wilson, 2007)

"An estimated 80% of North Americans suffer from Adrenal Fatigue at some point in their lives. Sometimes this is temporary and only lasts a few days. At other times it can be debilitating and last for years (or a lifetime if nothing is done about it)."

Dr. Wilson coined the term "adrenal fatigue" in 1998 to identify a group of signs and symptoms that people experience as a result of suboptimal adrenal function. Although it affects millions of people in the United States and around the world, conventional medicine does not yet recognize it as a distinct syndrome.

As adrenal function declines, organs and body systems are progressively and profoundly affected. Changes occur in carbohydrate, protein and fat metabolism; fluid and electrolyte balance; heart and cardiovascular system; and even sex drive levels.

Typical symptoms include fatigue, anxiety, nervousness, bone loss, increased abdominal fat, high blood sugar, allergies/asthma, arthritis, sleep disturbances, memory lapses, sugar cravings, chemical sensitivities and low energy.

How Can You Tell If Your Adrenals Are Fatigued?

- You feel tired for no reason.
- You have trouble getting up in the morning, even when you go to bed at a reasonable hour.
- You are feeling rundown or overwhelmed.
- You have difficulty bouncing back from stress or illness.
- You crave salty and sweet snacks.
- You feel more awake, alert and energetic after 6 pm than you do all day.

Most saliva hormone tests can uncover biochemical imbalances that can be underlying causes of such conditions as chronic stress, adrenal fatigue, anxiety, chronic fatigue, obesity, diabetes, depression, insomnia and many other chronic conditions.

The National Institutes of Health (NIH) and the World Health Organization (WHO) recognize saliva cortisol testing as being very accurate. Some insurance plans also cover saliva cortisol testing. Labs such as ZRT Lab (www.salivatest.com) allow patients to order tests directly.

Dr. Wilson's Recommended Food Choices

The food choices you make are essential to your health, especially when suffering from adrenal fatigue. By eating natural, high-quality food at frequent, regular intervals, you can help avoid drops in blood sugar and boost adrenal health and energy levels.

One of the major dietary mistakes made by people with low adrenal output is not eating soon enough after waking. It is very important to eat before 10:00 am; between 11:00 am and 11:30 am for lunch; a nutritious snack between 2:00 pm to 3 pm; and your evening meal between 5 and 6 pm. A high-quality snack before bed can help sleep disturbances.

What To Eat & Drink Summary from Dr. Wilson

1) Eat a wide variety of whole, natural foods
2) Combine a healthy fat, protein and carbohydrate source with every meal
3) Eat lots of vegetables, especially the brightly colored ones
4) Salt your food to a pleasant taste
5) Eat mainly whole grains as your source of carbohydrate
6) Combine grains with legumes (beans), or legumes with seeds or nuts to form a complete protein
7) Avoid fruit in the morning
8) Mix 1-2 tablespoons of fresh essential oils (cold pressed olive, grape seed, etc.) into grains, vegetables and meats daily
9) Eat high-quality food

Ironically, foods made with sugar and white flour—donuts, rolls, pies, cakes, cookies, candy bars and soft drinks—are the ones many people experiencing adrenal fatigue crave the most. The problem is that they raise blood sugar, causing an excess insulin release. The excess insulin causes blood sugar levels to crash, often leading to hypoglycemic symptoms and more cravings, creating a dangerous cycle.

Beverages that help alleviate adrenal fatigue are water, green tea, barley tea, bancha tea, herbal teas, goat's milk, vegetable juice and carob. Avoid chocolate, caffeine, alcohol and soft drinks.

Are you one of those people who struggle to wake up every day and only after a pot of coffee or two soda pops do you feel like you can finally start to function? Maybe you find your brain just doesn't engage like it used to. Fatigue is at almost epidemic levels in the United States. Half of all adults seeking medical treatment complain of fatigue.

There are foods that energize and foods that calm; it has only been in the last decade that research has been able to explain why. Our feelings, mood and energy levels are in a large part controlled by neurons—nerve cells in the brain that communicate by use of chemical messengers called neurotransmitters. Studies have shown that changes in the levels of neurotransmitters dopamine and norepinephrine dramatically affect energy levels, which is why they are called "wake up" chemicals. These chemicals allow us to think more clearly, be more motivated and have more energy.

Our diet should provide us with the raw materials needed for the production of neurotransmitters. What we eat or don't eat can have a large effect on how we feel. The building blocks for neurotransmitters are amino acids. There are 25 known amino acids. They are essential for growth and repair of body tissue, hormone production, enzymes, antibodies and brain chemistry and help transport other chemicals throughout the body. Amino acids come from protein; not all protein sources are high in all the various amino acids. The building block for norepinephrine and dopamine is tyrosine; this essential amino acid is found in fish, chicken, turkey and yogurt.

The best quality protein foods are free-range lamb, free-range beef, cold water fish, beans, free-range eggs, lentils, quinoa, free-range chicken and seeds like pumpkin, sesame and almond. You will note I did not mention dairy; it should be used sparingly and not as a staple. Research has shown that Americans consume more dairy than any other country in the world and we have the highest rate of osteoporosis and fractures. It may be because our dairy is pasteurized and commercially farmed. If the cattle aren't healthy, then the foods that they produce won't be, either.

How much protein do you need? The easiest measure is the palm of your hand. Your daily intake should roughly be the size of your palm (about 3-5 ounces depending on if you are male or female).[188]

Another cause of fatigue is low iron levels. Iron is essential for energy. This is particularly true for women in the perimenopausal (30-50) age group. The best source of iron is organ meats (like liver) and red meat. But not everyone likes liver, and some may be on reduced red meat diets, so what other foods are available? Try pumpkin seeds, strawberries, molasses, spirulina, parsley, watercress, cumin and sesame seeds. For best bioavailability, be sure you have plenty of vitamin C in your diet as well. The best lab test to have is a serum ferritin test—not an iron test. If your ferritin levels are low, you may not only feel tired all the time but your hair may be thinning and your thyroid sluggish.

To prevent afternoon energy slumps, try eating a lunch that contains healthy protein like a hardboiled egg, half of a chicken breast or salmon. Foods like potatoes, pastas or rice can leave you feeling sleepy or muddled because they stimulate the neurotransmitter tryptophan which jump-starts the production of serotonin, which can be calming and sedative.

Moderate coffee intake. Not only is it a diuretic but it can be a significant energy drain when consumed daily in large quantities. Added sugars and caffeine drain the adrenal glands, trace minerals and vitamins from your body.

Now Let's Hear It For The Men

Andropause

Andropause has been called the Male Menopause. I first started studying more about this subject when a 50-year-old client said to me, "If I'd known turning fifty was a door slamming shut on my life, I would have never turned it." He was successful and relatively healthy but feeling insecure, frustrated and depressed. I asked myself, Why?

Between the ages of 40 and 55, men can begin experiencing a phenomenon similar to the female menopause, called andropause. Unlike women, men do not have a clear-cut signpost such as the cessation of menstruation and hot flashes to mark this transition, but both are distinguished by a drop in hormone levels: progesterone

---

[188] (Sally Fallon & Mary Enig, 2001)

and sometimes estrogens in the female, testosterone in the male. In men, the changes occur gradually and may be accompanied by changes in attitudes and moods, fatigue, a loss of energy, and decreased sex drive and physical agility.

Starting at about age 30, testosterone levels in men drop by about 10 percent every decade. At the same time, another factor in the body called sex hormone binding globulin, or SHBG, is increasing. SHBG traps much of the testosterone that is still circulating and makes it unavailable to exert its effects in the body's tissues. What is left over does the beneficial work and is known as "bioavailable" testosterone.

Studies show this decline in testosterone can put men at risk for other health problems like heart disease, diabetes, depression, muscle loss/weakness, high blood pressure, elevated cholesterols, phantom joint and muscle pain, slowed healing, increased cancer risks, mild to moderate weight gain, prolonged fatigue and osteoporosis. Since this can coincide with a life stage when many men begin to question their values, accomplishments and direction in life, it's often difficult to realize the changes occurring are related to more than just external conditions. Attitude, psychological stress, alcohol, smoking, injuries, surgery, medications, obesity and infections can contribute to its onset.

Testosterone has a profound effect on brain chemistry in both men and women. This dramatic change in brain chemistry can affect one's marriage, friendships and other relationships. For some people, it can lead to alcohol or drug abuse problems.

Getting The Answers

Andropause was first described in medical literature in the 1940s. Andropause went underdiagnosed and undertreated for decades because standard lab tests could not accurately assess hormone levels. There is also a widespread misunderstanding that hormonal problems affect only women.

Also, symptoms can be vague and vary among individuals. Men may not admit they have a problem and, if they do, their physicians may not think of low testosterone as a possible culprit. They may instead simply diagnose it as depression or a part of normal aging.

Salivary hormone testing from labs like ZRT Lab in Beaverton, Oregon, have only been available to men and women for the last few years. This form of testing allows health care providers to accurately diagnose hormone levels and design proper treatment protocols.

If you think that you may be experiencing andropause or would like more information on this subject, look for a qualified bio-identical hormone practitioner in your area.

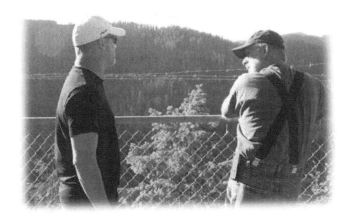

Turmeric

Turmeric (*Curcuma longa*) or Indian saffron has been used for centuries in India and Southeast Asia. In these areas, the prevalence of Alzheimer's disease and various cancers are much lower than they are in the United States and other Western countries.

Turmeric is a perennial plant native to India and cultivated in China, Bengal and Java for its rhizomes. Several other species of the curcuma genus grow wild in the forests of Southern Asia, including in India, Indonesia and Indochina, and in some Pacific Islands such as Hawaii. These cultures have used turmeric for culinary and medicinal purposes for millennia.

Turmeric is a mild aromatic stimulant used in the manufacture of curry powders and mustards. It is in the same family as ginger, cardamom and zedoary. The curcumin in turmeric has recently been shown to be effective against breast cancer, osteoporosis, gluten sensitivity, Alzheimer's disease, skin conditions and arthritis.

Scientific literature supports that this widely used spice possesses potent anti-inflammatory and antioxidant properties. However, curcumin is unable to be readily absorbed from dietary sources and does not produce adequate, sustained blood levels for optimal impact on its own. Use in combination with black pepper or dried ginger to help activate turmeric, or choose supplements that include them.

I encourage you to use turmeric in cooking, salad dressings, soups, rice dishes or sauces, as this is one of the most traditional ways of utilizing this herb. In the book

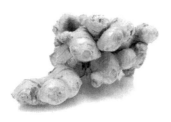

The Blue Zones it shows that the cultures with the greatest number of centenarians commonly use turmeric liberally in their diets. One interesting way is via goat milk.

The Science

In a recent study it was discovered that curcumin's natural anti-inflammatory and antioxidant properties may reduce both the oxidative damage and pathological changes that could lead to brain abnormalities. More precisely, curcumin has been

186

shown to decrease the incidence of harmful plaques by slowing deposition of beta-amyloid precursor protein (APP) within the brain, which is hypothesized to play a pivotal role in the progression of Alzheimer's disease.

Curcumin also benefits bones. Bone health and strength is a significant concern for people in the United States; it is estimated that 34 million people have low bone density and are at risk of further problems. Millions of Americans may be overdosing on calcium thinking it is helping their bones. Current nutrigenomics research supports the idea that our bones require a long list of nutrients to maintain their flexibility and strength. Sulphanes contained in turmeric are some of those vital nutrients.

The researchers concluded "curcumin can prevent further deterioration of the bone structure and produce beneficial changes in bone turnover (if you are not taking a prescription bone medication that prevents this). The change of inflammatory cytokines, including TNF-alpha and IL-6, may play a significant role in the mechanisms of action of curcumin, but the detailed mechanism remains unknown."

A recent study evaluated curcumin's effects on allergic airway inflammation and hyper-responsiveness. According to the American Academy of Allergy, Asthma and Immunology, 34.1 million Americans have been diagnosed with asthma during their lifetime, and the academy estimates that the number of Americans with asthma will increase by over 100 million by 2025. The study authors stated that in mice, "Curcumin attenuates the development of allergic airway inflammation and hyper-responsiveness, possibly through inhibition of NF-kappaB activation in the asthmatic lung tissue. Our results indicate that curcumin may attenuate the development of asthma by inhibition of NF-kappaB activation."

So, add a little spice to your life and help out your bones, brain and lungs!

Curcurmin Common Uses

- Abrasions/cuts
- Aches and pains
- Cancer prevention
- Candida/yeast infection
- Cholesterol control
- Concentration/memory
- Eye care/vision
- Gout
- Heart tonics
- Lupus
- Osteoarthritis
- Rheumatoid arthritis
- Smoking cessation

Properties

- Anti-inflammatory
- Analgesic
- Antibacterial
- Cardiac tonic
- Hepatic
- COX-2 inhibitor
- Antifungal

Constituents

- Volatile oils (terpene, curcumen)
- Starch
- Albumen (30%)
- Coloring due chiefly to curcumin
- Potassium
- Vitamin C

NSAIDs: A Cautionary Tale

Millions of Americans routinely take over-the-counter medications known as NSAIDs (nonsteroidal anti-inflammatory drugs), namely:

- Ibuprofen (e.g. brand names Advil™, Motrin™, Nuprin™)
- Naproxen (e.g. brand names Aleve™, Naprosyn™)
- COX-2 inhibitors (e.g. brand name Celebrex™)

NSAIDs comprise a large class of drugs used to reduce inflammation and relieve pain. In addition to aspirin, there are currently several types of both non-prescription (over-the-counter) NSAIDs and prescription brands of NSAIDs. These medications do not come with a red warning label which would alert the consumer to the potential dangers.

NSAIDs are known to damage kidney and liver function in some individuals. On April 9, 2014, physician news site Medscape posted that NSAIDs are linked to higher atrial fibrillation risk:

"Taking nonsteroidal anti-inflammatory (NSAID) drugs appears to be associated with an increased risk for atrial fibrillation (AF), even after adjustment for ventricular end-diastolic dimension, known to be increased with NSAID use, a new study confirms.

"Patients using NSAIDs for 2 to 4 weeks had a 76% higher risk of developing AF compared with those who hadn't taken these pain medications, researchers found.

"The underlying mechanism connecting NSAID use with AF isn't clear and 'deserves further attention,' the authors conclude. AF, a common arrhythmia in the elderly, is associated with stroke, heart failure, increased mortality and reduced life expectancy. NSAID use has also been related to myocardial infarction, stroke and heart failure. Other recent studies have suggested that NSAID use may increase the risk for AF, the researchers note."

Millions of people use these medications regularly. I use them myself on occasion, but I always increase my water consumption when taking them to reduce potential kidney damage.

If you have a history of heart problems or kidney disease please speak with a knowledgeable pharmacist and your healthcare provider before continuing to take NSAIDs.

Natural Pain Relievers

There are many herbs and foods that reduce inflammation. However, they may take longer to take effect and the quantity needed is higher than a once-daily prescription medication. Some individuals may need to continue prescription anti-inflammatories, but with the incorporation of natural therapies such as Boswellia serrata, turmeric, Una de Gato, MSM and proteolytic enzymes, medication dosages may be reduced.

Boswellia serrata, also known as Indian frankincense, is a tree native to the mountainous regions of the Middle East and is related to the tree that yields the frankincense referenced in the Bible. Its trunk is slashed to permit the flow of a resinous gum, which is also known as Guggulu and locally called *shallaki* (Sanskrit).

After collection, the resin is cured in specialized bamboo baskets before being broken into pieces and graded according to color and shape. Boswellia serrata has a very pleasant, exotic scent when burned as incense alone or in combination with other resins.

The gum oleoresin consists of essential oils, gum and terpenoids. The terpenoid portion contains the boswellic acids that have been shown to be the active constituents in Boswellia. Today, extracts are typically standardized to contain 37.5–65% boswellic acids.

Boswellia has been shown to be as efficient and, in many cases, better than drugs like Phenylbutazone and other anti-inflammatory medications. Boswellia serrata gum resin is widely used in Ayurvedic formulations for treating asthma and arthritis.

So before you pop another Advil™ or Aleve™ for the pain in your back, consider your options. Increase your consumption of mineral waters which help improve kidney function. Reduce inflammatory foods, including polyunsaturated oils, and try Boswellia for pain relief. This herb has no known side effects, and it is safe for dogs as well.

Traditional Herbs To The Rescue

Often we catch a cold because our immune systems have been worn down by poor eating habits, stress, long hours and overindulging. This may be one of the reasons so many folks come down with colds following the holiday season. Most of us simply need to rest and drink lots of fluids.

Every traditional culture possesses a vast pharmacopeia of herbs to help the body fight off foreign invaders. This natural pharmacy has been relegated to the realm of "quacks and oddballs" over the last five decades and replaced with trendy designer drugs. But the side effects of these drugs can open up a Pandora's box of health challenges. They also, for the most part, do not cure but simply suppress symptoms. Herbs can help build natural resistance through nutrients, vitamins, phytochemicals, tannins and a host of ingredients that we are not even aware of yet.

Viruses do not become resistant to herbs like they do to commonly prescribed medications, many of which are intended for bacterial infections. Herbs strengthen the immune system without killing the beneficial flora that resides in the digestive system. Remember that 85% of your immune system is in your digestive tract. Overuse of antibiotics can lead to side effects and drug-resistant microbes.

Here are some ways to boost your natural immunity:

- Take **probiotics** (healthy live bacterium) every day for your digestive system. Probiotics are currently being studied for their benefits for cancer patients and those with chronic illness.
- Take high-quality **digestive enzymes** before every meal or at the very least, twice daily. Enzymes are key players in immune function. Years ago I was told by Dr. Udo Erasmus to take digestive enzymes every hour, just like some folks do with vitamin C, when coming down with a cold. This boosts viral defense mechanisms without the gastric upset so common with vitamin C.
- The oil from **oregano** leaf helps eliminate bacteria and fungi, particularly in the gastrointestinal tract. Research suggests that oregano oil inhibits unfriendly parasites, fungi and yeasts.
- **Garlic** is widely researched in the United States and abroad and is one of the most revered botanical foods. Garlic strengthens the immune system by working against immune invaders and attacking bacteria, viruses, fungi and parasites. Use fresh in broths and add liberally to vegetables and meats. Always use fresh garlic, not dried or canned.
- **Grapefruit seed** extract is antibacterial, antimicrobial, antiseptic, antiviral, antifungal and antiparasitic. Of all herbs, it is perhaps the only true antibiotic.
- **Mullein** has long been used in herbal medicine, especially in remedies that aim to soothe the respiratory tract. [189] Remedies involve the use of mullein's flowers and leaves. In test-tube research, mullein has been found to fight flu-causing viruses.
- **Horehound** has used internally to treat upper respiratory congestion, whooping cough, bronchitis, asthma, tuberculosis and diarrhea. This herb is intended for short-term use and some medications may interact. A strong tea taken twice daily for two to three days is all you will likely need. It tastes awful, but it works!
- **Chili peppers** can be used liberally in foods, especially in soups. Chilies have high natural vitamin C content and act as a vasodilator, opening blood vessels.

---

[189] https://www.herb-pharm.com/products/product-detail/mullein-blend

- **Gypsy Cold Care®** tea (available in most natural food stores) is handy to have at work when the first symptoms are apparent. Also, try Throat Coat® and Breath Easy®.
- **Ginger** is used as an antioxidant; to help prevent motion and morning sickness; and to relieve sore throat, nausea, vomiting and headaches.
- **Peppermint** helps to soothe an upset stomach and open airways. Adding this to the horehound herb tea will help improve the flavor.

Last, but far from least, is the warm healing benefits of homemade chicken soup. Researchers have found that the fat from organically raised chickens is one of the reasons it is so beneficial for getting rid of a cold or flu bug. Combine this with garlic, celery, carrots, onion, mushrooms, chilies, rosemary, sage, oregano and thyme and you have the makings for a rich soup that heals the body.

If you are prone to chest and head congestion, I advise you to avoid eggs and dairy during the cooler months as they encourage the production of mucous and phlegm. Gluten can also cause congestion in some individuals.

Hawthorn, An Herb Worthy Of Consideration

Hawthorn is a tall-growing shrub that bears white flowers, red berries and large vicious thorns. Some believe the thorns were used to weave the crown that Christ wore at the crucifixion.[190]

"The use of hawthorn dates back to Dioscorides. Native Americans, Europeans and Chinese people have long used the hawthorn shrub, including its fruit, leaves, and flowers, as a remedy for health problems." *(webmd.com/vitamins-and-supplements/hawthorn-uses-and-risks, 2015)*

The plant gained widespread popularity in European and American herbal medicine only toward the end of the 19th century. Hawthorn preparations remain popular in Europe and have gained some acceptance in the U.S.

Studies have shown that hawthorn can normalize both high and low blood pressure. According to WebMD,"In one study that combined the results of earlier studies on people with heart failure, hawthorn extract was linked to fewer symptoms of heart failure. People taking hawthorn had less fatigue and shortness of breath.

---

[190] Natural-Medicinal-Herbs.com/herbs/hawthorn.htm, 2015

"Another study indicated that people with type 2 diabetes who took hawthorn extract for four months had a drop in diastolic blood pressure (the bottom number in a blood pressure reading)."

Note that hawthorn can interact with many types of blood pressure medications. Make sure you consult with a knowledgeable herbalist and let your integrative cardiologist or doctor know you are using hawthorn.

Most of the beneficial actions of hawthorn are attributable to its flavanols, oligomeric proanthocyanidins (OPCs), although in clinical trials hawthorn has proven most effective when the whole berries are used, rather than isolated constituents from them. *(Hawthorn, 2009)*

Hawthorn has been used over the centuries to prevent and treat arrhythmias, heart attack, hypertension, congestive heart disease, stroke, colitis and diarrhea, and to improve oxygen utilization in the heart muscle.

OPCs are highly beneficial in the prevention and reversal of atherosclerosis (by inhibiting the histidine decarboxylase enzyme which catalyzes the excessive conversion of histidine to histamine that is usually observed in atherosclerosis patients and by inhibiting the oxidation of LDL cholesterol). Additionally OPCs inhibit some aspects of the aging process (by enhancing the body's renewal of collagen and inhibiting excessive cross-linking).

Research has shown that OPCs help in the healing and prevention of "gastric ulcers by inhibiting the excessive production of histamine within the gastric mucosa by the histidine decarboxylase enzyme."

OPCs also benefit the eyes, brain and skin. OPCs are found in high levels in some 'super foods'.

"The term *proanthocyanidins* is derived as follows pro=before, anthocyanins=red, referring to their colorless property and their ability to be transformed into (red) Anthocyanins." *(General Health Benefits of OPC Pycnogenol Super Anti Oxidant ... (n.d.). Retrieved from http://www.allergydiets.com/opcgeneraloverview.html_br)*

OPCs, found in hawthorn and other plants, is a vital nutrient for the heart and circulatory system. Once again, modern science is validating what historical herbalists learned via observation and oral tradition: hawthorn improves the structural integrity of collagen and lowers serum cholesterol.

Traditional herbalists report that the protective effects of hawthorn berries, flowers and leaves are achieved after long-term use. It usually takes one to two months before the effects of hawthorn become noticeable. It can be safely used for long periods of time without the risk of toxicity or side effects.

Hawthorn fruit can be eaten as food. The fruits are also canned and processed into jam, candy and drinks. According to Monica Shaw, haws (the berry) "should be picked late in the season (October and November are ideal), when they are as ripe as possible. Although hawthorn berries come off the tree easily, they often bring with them lots of stems which should be removed before cooking—a slightly time-consuming process. On their own, haw berries aren't anything exciting—they're mostly pip and taste a bit like a dry, under-ripe apple. They really need to be cooked to get anything useful out of them."(Shaw)[191, 192, 193]

[191] www.antiagingdoctor.co.za
[192] www.sensitivefoods.com/opcgeneraloverview.html
[193] www.greatbritishchefs.com

Magnesium

Magnesium has been called the most important mineral for human beings and all living organisms. It is critical to the metabolic process of one-celled organisms and is the second most abundant mineral found in human cells. Magnesium is involved in all aspects of cell production and growth. In both plants and animals, magnesium is involved in hundreds of enzyme processes promoting life and health.

Currently, 17 minerals are considered essential for human life. As with most minerals, magnesium naturally combines with other elements. By combining with sulfur, magnesium makes Epsom salts; magnesium combined with carbon makes magnesium carbonate; and it combines with calcium to make dolomite. Like calcium, magnesium is alkalizing, reducing acidosis (high acid).

Approximately 60% of the body's total magnesium is concentrated in the bones, 20% is in muscles, and 20% is in soft tissues and the liver. Magnesium works inside our tissue cells, producing ATP energy and triggering the production of the body's protein structures by producing DNA.

What Does Magnesium Do?

- Magnesium is a cofactor, assisting enzymes in chemical reactions, including temperature regulation.
- Magnesium transports energy.
- Magnesium is necessary for the synthesis of protein.
- Magnesium transports nerve signals.
- Magnesium relaxes muscles.

Calcium and magnesium are interrelated; neither can act without eliciting a reaction from the other and they are antagonistic towards one another. Enzymes that depend on sufficient amounts of intracellular magnesium will be detrimentally affected by small increases in cellular calcium. If too much calcium is present in the cellular tissue, cell division, growth and intermediary metabolism are adversely affected. Magnesium causes calcium to dissolve in the body, enabling the blood to take it up and transport it. If you are not receiving adequate amounts of magnesium and you are supplementing with calcium, you may be increasing your risk factors for heart disease, muscle spasms, fibromyalgia, dental cavities and kidney stones.

Current research has identified that calcium supplementation in men may increase their prostate cancer risks by 38%. Calcium supplementation recommendations for women have been dropped to 600 mg daily to prevent arterial occlusion.

All muscles, including the heart and blood vessels, are affected if magnesium is deficient. Calcium floods the smooth muscle cells causing spasms and constricted blood flow. This can lead to high blood pressure, arterial spasms, angina and heart attack.

Supplemental magnesium should be taken at a different time of the day to supplementary calcium (as calcium prevents the absorption of magnesium if it is consumed in conjunction with magnesium).

The absorption of magnesium decreases rapidly when more than 200 mg is consumed at one time. It is therefore advisable to take magnesium supplements in divided doses during the day. Many of the therapeutic benefits associated with magnesium are optimized when magnesium is consumed as magnesium aspartate and combined with potassium aspartate. High dietary levels of phosphorus (found in soda pop) inhibit the body's absorption of magnesium. All processed foods and beverages are devoid of magnesium.

Poor digestion and low stomach acid can lead to magnesium deficiency, as can stress, advanced age, arthritis, diabetes, gallbladder disease, osteoporosis, asthma and depression. One of the most common over-the-counter drugs are antacids; heartburn and indigestion are the result of bad eating choices and taking acid reducers limits the amount of acid available for the digestion of essential minerals like magnesium. Calcium carbonate antacids deplete already deficient reserves of magnesium, increasing the likelihood of insomnia, restless leg and chronic health challenges.

Health Challenges that Benefit from Optimum Magnesium Intake

Anxiety & panic attacks	Detoxification
Asthma	Diabetes
Blood clots	Fatigue
Bowel disease	Heart disease
Cystitis	Hypertension
Depression	Hypoglycemia

Insomnia
Kidney disease
Migraine
Musculoskeletal health
Nerve health

Gynecological health
Osteoporosis
Raynaud's syndrome
Tooth decay

Salt For Life

The media and mainsntream medical establishment derided salt for decades, claiming that it leads to heart disease. In these reports, there was often no differentiation made between refined table salt and other types of salt.

Salt was historically a very valuable commodity. Entire civilizations developed around the salt industry and trade. Salzburg, a city in Austria, is named after salt. Roman soldiers were paid in salt, leading to the expression "he's not worth his salt". The earliest known writings about salt occurred 5,000 years ago in China. Ancient Egyptians recorded salt production in paintings. Salt is so important to life, animals will travel great distances to get to it.

Sixty percent of the body's sodium is stored in the fluids surrounding the cell; 10% is stored inside the cell. Sodium is the principal negatively charged ion in our cells responsible for the conduction and regulation of electricity (energy); it is the primary electrolyte. Some clinicians believe salt is alkalizing, thus reducing acidosis. Dr. David Brownstein, MD, has found that many individuals with high blood pressure improve when they switch to unrefined salt.

The body is 70% water and the brain is 80% water. An adult contains about 250 grams of salt and a baby contains 14 grams. Water and salt are necessary for metabolism and detoxification as well as for hormone, immune and nervous system function.

A connection between salt and hypertension was first discovered in 1904. Animal studies done over the next fifty years supported the hypothesis. However, no one looked at the amount of salt given to the animals and the form of salt used.

Facts about Salt

- People who crave salt are often found to be suffering from adrenal insufficiency.
- Sodium may alleviate constipation.
- Sodium sulfate may alleviate diarrhea.
- Nausea, vomiting and flatulence may occur as a result of sodium deficiency.
- Optimal (but not excessive) sodium levels are required for the correct function of the kidneys.
- Sodium deficiency may cause blurred vision.
- Optimal sodium levels are required for the correct function of the lymphatic system (sodium is a component of lymph).
- 30% of the body's sodium concentrates in the bones.
- Correct potassium-sodium balance is essential for the correct function of the muscles; shrinkage of the muscles can occur as a result of sodium deficiency. Sodium may facilitate proper muscle contraction. Muscle cramps may occur as a result of sodium deficiency.

Not All Salt Is Good For You

The type of salt used in commercial foods is not a health food. It is processed via chemicals that are used to clean and purify the salt from all contaminants but also strip out minerals. Salt naturally isn't white, nor does it flow easily; this is the result of chemical processing.

Some of the chemicals used in salt refining are sulfuric acid, chlorine, anti-caking agents like sodium ferrocyanide, ammonium citrate, aluminum silicates and dextrose. Unrefined sea salt from companies like Celtic Sea Salt may contain over 80 key and trace minerals. Key and trace minerals are essential to health; they are the foundation of every biochemical response in the body. Standard table salt is straight sodium chloride, and although it may have added iodine along with the aforementioned chemicals.

Celtic sea salt can be useful in the detoxification of harmful chemicals from the body. Bromine is one such chemical found in processed foods and drinks like Mountain Dew. Bromine bumps iodine off of cell receptor sites affecting healthy thyroid function. People who ingest enough bromine feel dull, apathetic and have difficulty concentrating, may have headaches, depression and irritability. Bromine has also been linked to breast cancer. Salt competes with bromine in the kidneys for re-absorption, a low-salt diet allows for greater amounts of bromine to be absorbed. .

Mark Bitterman and his family have created a wonderful shop called The Meadow in Portland, Oregon, that sells a tantalizing array of salts. Mark is the author of *Salted, A Manifesto on the World's Most Essential Mineral, with Recipes*. I was delighted to add it to my collection and recommend it to nutritionists, foodies and chefs.

Mankind, like animals, must have salt to survive. It is necessary for heart, thyroid, liver, brain and stomach function. But the industrialized salt commonly used in the United States is very different than that extracted from the salt mines in Asia and Europe.

Natural salt comes in a variety of colors, flavors and crystal characteristics. Some are perfectly suited for confectionary masterpieces like *fleur de sel* caramels. These salted caramels originated in Brittany, France, due to the availability of the artisan-made salts in the region.

In the United States, we generally use three varieties of salt, made much the same way. As Mark Bitterman writes, "Some things do not belong in our food supply. Industrial salts like cheap sea salt, kosher salt and table salt are products that few people want in their kitchens if they understand and face up to how they are made."

If we are enjoying produce from CSAs, farmers' markets and home and community gardens, we already know how much better local fresh foods taste than limp lifeless store-bought versions. So why wouldn't we want to use natural salts to make those flavors pop and zing even more?

Iodine, The Forgotten Mineral

Approximately 1.5 billion people, one-third of the global population, are at risk of iodine deficiency as defined by the World Health Organization (WHO). Iodine deficiency has been identified as a significant public health problem in 129 countries. Iodine deficiency can result in mental retardation, goiter, increased child and infant mortality, infertility, hypothyroidism, impaired immune function, fibrocystic breasts, and cancers of the thyroid, breast, prostate, endometrium, ovaries and uterus. The WHO has recognized that iodine deficiency is the world's greatest single cause of preventable mental retardation.

Iodine is a relatively rare element found primarily in sea water and sea foods like kelp and fish (cod, sea bass, haddock and perch). Seaweed is the most abundant source of iodine; this algae concentrates the iodine found in ocean water. Kelp, however, also concentrates large quantities of contaminants and chemicals like perchlorate (rocket fuel), fluoride and bromine.

Every cell in the body utilizes iodine. The thyroid gland contains a higher concentration of iodine than any other organ in the body. Large amounts of iodine are also stored in the salivary glands, spinal fluid, gastric mucosa, breasts, ovaries, prostate and the body of the eye.

A Little History

Bernard Courtois discovered iodine in 1811 while making gunpowder. When he added sulphuric acid (made from seaweed) to his mixture, a purple vapor appeared (*iodes* is Greek for violet). Iodine was first used medically in 1824 by Jean-Baptiste Boussingault; he found that the iodine-rich water found at silver mining sites prevented goiter. In the early 1900s, goiter was prevalent in the states bordering the Great Lakes. In 1924, a study in the state of Michigan showed that 40% of the school-age children had enlarged thyroid glands. Iodized salt was introduced to counter this and by 1928 a 75% reduction in goiter was observed. The WHO actively promotes the use of iodized salt for the prevention of goiter.

Why Are We Low In Iodine?

You may think that iodized salt has eliminated deficiencies in the United States, but the data does not support this conclusion. Studies done by the National Health and Nutrition Examination Survey over the last 30 years show that levels of iodine have dropped by over 50 percent. This is occuring across all demographics, regardless of ethnicity, region, economic status and race.

Refined salt does not provide the most bioavailable form of iodine. Foods such as bread can more effectively raise serum iodine levels, but this changed in the 1980s when iodine was replaced with bromide in flour and baked goods and the population was encouraged to go on low-salt diets.

Bromide is in the halide family and all halides (fluoride, chloride, bromide, iodine) compete for absorption and receptor sites. Bromide is a toxic substance that has no therapeutic use in the human body. Perchlorate is a man-made substance. Perchlorate contamination of water supplies is widespread and is another reason that iodine levels are dropping.

Individuals of northern European ancestry seem to be more prone to iodine deficiency. This is primarily due to a generational deficiency resulting from changes in farming practices. In the past in coastal areas of England, Wales, Ireland, Scotland, Scandinavia and France, it was a common practice to collect seaweed and spread it on the fields for fertilizer. This added the essential iodine back into the soil for the grain crops, which in turn fed the animals and the population.

Iodine Loading Test

This test is used to assess whole body sufficiency for the essential element iodine. Orthoiodosupplementation is the daily amount of the essential element iodine needed for whole body sufficiency. The test consists of ingesting four tablets of a solid dosage form of Lugol (Iodoral®) containing a total of 50 mg of iodine/iodide.

Currently, there are two laboratories performing the iodine/iodide loading test that I trust:
- Labrix Clinical Services Inc. in Oregon City, OR
- ZRT Lab in Portland, OR

Ferritin: Overlooked Biologically Available Iron

Over the last five years our office has requested ferritin serum levels on about one-third of our clients. Some individuals with unexplained body and muscle pain had very high ferritin levels and others who were low in ferritin were short of breath, irritable and suffered from low-grade headaches or elevated TSH (thyroid test) levels without deficiencies in free T3 or free T4.

In my opinion, ferritin and iron levels are being overlooked in many individuals. Common thinking is that iron levels are only low in menstruating women, cancer patients and those with blood diseases.

Ferritin is a protein found inside cells that stores iron until it is needed. A ferritin test indirectly measures the amount of iron in your blood. The amount of ferritin in your blood (serum ferritin level) is directly related to the amount of iron stored in your body.[194] While iron stores and iron levels may be reflected in a standard CBC (complete blood count) or Chem panel, by the time low ferritin levels are reflected the client may have been without adequate iron for years.

---

[194] www.nlm.nih.gov/medlineplus/ency/article/003490.htm

This was the case with one 45-year-old female whose low iron levels had been overlooked by her primary care provider. Since her youth she suffered from weakness, heart palpitations, irritability, low grade headaches and mild restless leg symptoms. Antidepressants and pain medications were the solutions offered by her medical provider.

Elderly clients may be told they are anemic based solely on their CBC panels, as was the case with one client in her 70s who had a family history of hemochromatosis. For years she had suffered from arthritic symptoms; her doctors recommended NSAIDs. On closer evaluation, her ferritin levels were found to be 1790 (normal range is 12-500). This level indicated that she was unable to convert iron into hemoglobin, has liver or kidney disease,[195] or has had a cardiac event causing the release of ferritin into the bloodstream. Her doctor prescribed her iron supplements and told her to improve her diet.

Ferritin levels are not revealed in a standard CBC lab test. Low ferritin may be a widespread problem overlooked by providers.[196,197,198,199]

Ferritin is stored in the bone marrow, intestinal wall, liver and spleen. You can have normal or even optimal serum iron and saturation levels and normal hemoglobin and hematocrit and still have low ferritin. Low ferritin levels can be caused by genetic conditions, celiac disease, anti-inflammatory medication use, or bacteria and viruses (they feed on iron).

The Linus Pauling Institute has stated that in addition to carrying oxygen in the blood, ferritin (iron) is an essential part of hundreds of proteins needed for energy, the synthesis of DNA and antioxidant enzymes. Low ferritin is a potentially serious condition.

[195] Biomarkers for Assessing and Managing Iron Deficiency Anemia in Late-Stage Chronic Kidney Disease: Future Research Needs: Identification of Future Research Needs From Comparative Effectiveness Review No. 83 [Internet].
Chung M, Chan JA, Moorthy D, Hadar N, Ratichek SJ, Concannon TW, Lau J.Rockville (MD): Agency for Healthcare Research and Quality (US); 2013 Jan.PMID:23762920[PubMed]
[196] http://www.nlm.nih.gov/medlineplus/ency/article/003490.htm
[197] What Causes Low Ferritin? Mar 7, 2011 | By Sandi Busch
[198] NIH/National Institute of Child Health and Human Development (NICHD) (2013, February 17). Lack of iron regulating protein contributes to high blood pressure of the lungs. *ScienceDaily*. Retrieved July 1, 2013, from http://www.sciencedaily.com /releases/2013/02/130217165414.htm
[199] Imperial College London (2011, December 16). Low iron levels in blood raises blood clot risk, new research suggests. ScienceDaily. Retrieved July 1, 2013, from http://www.sciencedaily.com- /releases/2011/12/111215095459.htm

Low ferritin can be asymptomatic. It is a precursor to anemia, as revealed by labs (saturation and serum iron). Symptoms of anemia mimic hypothyroidism: depression, achiness, fatigue, weakness, increased heart rate, palpitations, loss of sex drive, hair loss and foggy thinking. A patient may mistakenly believe they are having heart problems or need more thyroid medication. Excessively low ferritin as well as low iron make it difficult to control thyroid and adrenal health problems.

Low iron levels slow the conversion of T4 to T3. Biologically, insufficient iron levels may be affecting the first two of three steps of thyroid hormone synthesis by reducing the activity of the enzyme *thyroid peroxidase* which is dependent on iron. Low iron levels can increase circulating concentrations of TSH (thyroid stimulating hormone).

Iron is needed for the production of cortisol via the adrenal cortex. An iron-containing protein is present in high amounts in the adrenal cortex and is involved in the synthesis of corticosterone. Therefore, low iron can potentially lower cortisol levels, inducing adrenal fatigue.[200]

Note that iron stored as ferritin is incapable of initiating free radical reactions. Ferritin, therefore, inhibits the ability of iron to cause some types of cardiovascular diseases.

Low ferritin levels may increase the risk of fibromyalgia and restless legs syndrome (RLS); patients are often found to have significantly lower ferritin levels than healthy subjects.[201]

The World Health Organization estimates that as much as 80% of the world's population may be iron deficient. Many people in North America do not consume enough iron in their diet. Dietary iron comes in two chemical forms: heme and nonheme. Heme iron comes from flesh foods, primarily red meat. The iron from plant sources is nonheme and is roughly 10% bioavailable. Legumes, grains and rice are plant sources of iron, but they contain phytic acid which decreases the iron absorption by as much as 50 percent.

Antacids, milk thistle, anti-inflammatory medications, black tea and dairy products (including whey protein) can decrease ferritin levels and exacerbate malabsorption illnesses such as ulcerative colitis, IBS, Crohn's disease, celiac disease, GI ulcers and

---

[200] http://www.stopthethyroidmadness.com/ferritin/
[201] In-Tele-Health © 2009 (from Hyperhealth Pro CD-ROM)

colon cancer. Low ferritin can also cause excessive blood loss from menstruation and surgery.

Excessive stored iron (ferritin) was once believed to be a risk factor for cardiovascular diseases including atherosclerosis and heart attack. More recently, researchers have shown serum ferritin levels become elevated as a result of (not as a precursor to) inflammatory processes that lead to cardiovascular diseases. In other words, pre-existing cardiovascular disease most likely accounted for the high serum ferritin levels in the original study. Several scientific studies since have found no correlation between elevated ferritin levels and cardiovascular disease risk.[202, 203]

I frequently hear clients ask, "But why doesn't anyone tell you this? Why don't doctors look into this?"

First, no one knows your body and health better than you do. If you are exposed to information that empowers you to take back control of your health, and do so, the job of your primary health care provider just got easier, because you are doing your part to stay healthy, vibrant and productive.

Secondly, many health challenges have the same symptoms; this is one of the reasons why knowing your family history is important. Familial tendencies may give you a clue to what is causing your fatigue, heart palpitations, dizziness, shortness of breath or other symptoms associated with low ferritin. Low ferritin may also be a symptom of other health conditions like celiac disease, Crohn's disease and thyroid dysfunction. The key is to ensure that a deficiency like low ferritin is not overlooked so that health can be managed effectively.

What to do if ferritin is low? In order for your ferritin levels to read as low, a biologically iron-deficient state has to occur over a prolonged period. When reviewing lab results (depending on the lab) you will see ferritin ranges are 12-500 ng/mL or 15-400 ng/mL.[204, 205, 206] The thyroid and adrenal glands works best when ferritin is somewhere between 80-110 ng/mL. Women will routinely complain of hair loss between 40-60 ng/mL and fatigue and lightheadedness between 20-40 ng/mL; 20 ng/mL and lower can manifest in heart arrhythmias, breathlessness,

[202] In-Tele-Health ©2009 (from Hyperhealth Pro CD-ROM)
[203] Salonen, J. U., et al. High stored iron levels associated with excess risk of myocardial infarction in western Finnish men. Circulation. 86(3):803-811, 1992.
[204] http://www.stedmansonline.com/webFiles/Dict-Stedmans28/APP17.pdf
[205] https://www.labcorp.com/wps/portal/patient/healthlibrary
[206] https://www.labcorp.com/wps/portal/insurer/labcorpdifference

irritability, nerve pain and restless leg symptoms. Note that all of these symptoms can occur within what the lab results deem a normal range.

The very best food source of ferritin (iron) is liver, preferably pork liver. Liver is not commonly consumed in the United States. This cultural aversion to liver may account for the growing numbers of individuals low in not only iron but vitamin D and B12.[207, 208, 209, 210, 211]

Hem iron is the most bioavailable of the bound forms of iron. It is found mainly in flesh foods such as lean red meat, lamb, buffalo, wild game, sockeye salmon, tuna, pork and chicken legs. Next best sources are molasses, sesame seeds, pumpkin seeds, pistachios, dandelion, coco, rice bran, spirulina and cold water kelp.[212,213]

As we age, hydrochloric acid production diminishes. Many individuals take supplementary calcium to reduce the chance of osteoporosis as well as anti-inflammatory medications for osteoarthritis; both can interfere with ferritin. This, along with subpar nutritional intake, could increase the likelihood of low ferritin in elderly individuals and those living with chronic illness.

An early and accurate diagnosis may prevent unnecessary falls or medications, and ultimately lead to better quality of life.

[207] http://health.nytimes.com/health/guides/disease/anemia/risk-factors.html
[208] Stanford University (2005, April 6). Undiagnosed Anemia Common With Chronic Illness.
[209] [Guideline] American College of Obstetricians and Gynecologists (ACOG). Anemia in pregnancy. Jul 2008;[Full Text].

[212] http://www.nlm.nih.gov/medlineplus/ency/article/002422.htm
[213] In-Tele-Health © 2009 (from Hyperhealth Pro CD-ROM)

In the spring of 2010, I was introduced to Tom O'Bryan, DC, CCN, DACBN, and his compelling information on gluten sensitivity. I also poured through mountains of medical journal research supporting gluten as a leading cause of major illnesses. The information I learned has been invaluable in educating clients.

What Is Gluten & What Foods Contain It?

The proteins found in grains within the wheat family have toxic effects on the brain and body. Celiac disease, also called non-tropical sprue and gluten-sensitive enteropathy, is a hereditary condition in which a person has a delayed allergic reaction to gluten (a protein that causes dough to be sticky) found in cereals such as oats, wheat, barley and rye.

Gluten sensitivity and celiac disease are a potentially life-threatening, life-long condition.[214]

Gluten is a type of dietary protein; it is really a mixture of two proteins (the prolamine *gliadin* and the dietary protein *glutenin*) found in some cereal grains. The gliadin content of gluten is responsible for most of the toxic effects of gluten.

Gliadin is a type of prolamine—one of 35 found in wheat. These proteins create inflammation and gut permeability; as the delicate brushes called villi are worn away by gluten proteins, the immune system sends out armies called leukocytes to drive away invaders. Over time the immune system response to gluten erodes cells and tissues not only in the digestive tract but also in the brain, liver, bones, pancreas, heart and thyroid glands. The gut wall begins allowing partially digested foods to pass into the bloodstream. An individual may begin to feel weak, fatigued, and anemic, and experience body pain, headaches or allergies. The condition can lead to osteoporosis, elevated liver enzymes and other health problems.

One in three Americans of Northern European descent may have gluten sensitivity. There is a hereditary component to gluten intolerance. The incidence for first-line family members is two out of three. This quiet killer is prevalent today and is regularly featured in the *Journal of American Medicine*, the *American Journal of*

---

[214] (Lowell, 2005)

Hematology and the *New England Journal of Medicine*. Gluten sensitivity is relatively common in Ireland, Northern Europe and Italy.

There is an increased rate of malignancies (cancer) associated with celiac disease. The rates decline to normal levels after five years on a gluten-free therapeutic diet. The earlier the diagnosis and the sooner a patient can commence a gluten-free diet, the fewer autoimmune-type diseases the patient will acquire.

If left unaddressed, gut permeability can lead to thyroid illness, diabetes, osteoporosis, ADD/ADHD, ALS, MS, Parkinson's disease, neuropathies, muscle wasting and more.

Simply going gluten-free will not be enough to repair the damage done to the villi of the small intestine. Studies released in 2009 and early 2010 revealed that the small intestine, once damaged by gluten, develops a host of harmful bacteria such as streptococcus, neisseria, veillonella, gemellia, actinomyces, rothia and haemophillus. Additionally, researchers have found over 35 sequences of new bacteria in gluten sensitive patients' biopsies. Some feel these mutations or new bacteria are the result of genetically modified grains and the herbicides their cells have interfaced with.[215]

Here is a short list of the most common gluten-containing food ingredients:

Barley, bulgur, cereal binding, couscous, durum, einkorn, emmer, filler, farro, Graham flour, Kamut, malt, malt extract, malt flavoring, malt syrup, oat bran, oats, oat syrup, rye, semolina, spelt, triticale, wheat, wheat bran, wheat germ, wheat starch, hydrolyzed plant or vegetable protein (HPP/HVP), seasonings, flavorings, turkeys (may be injected with gluten for moistness or have gravy packets), starch, modified food starch, dextrin and maltodextrin.

Prescription and over-the-counter medications can contain gluten. Nutraceuticals can have gluten in the capsule or fillers and fiber supplements may contain wheat fiber and cellulose.

> **Note: Gluten and lactose are the most common fillers for medications**

---

[215] (Peter H. R Green, 2006)

Gluten can be found in thousands of everyday items including shampoo, gum, chocolate milk, fruit fillings, commercial soups, beer, lunch meats, syrups, soy sauce, ketchup, barbeque sauce, ice cream, non-dairy creamer and potato chips.

Many of us believe bread to be the staff of life. After all, the ancient Egyptians, Greeks and Romans cultivated wheat. Many clients don't want to accept that they may have an issue that could mean giving up breads, pasta, baked goods and pizza.

Agra-corporations have advanced the production of grain through hybridization and selective breeding, but also through sinister genetic splicing with genes from plants, chemicals and animals.

When a civilization can no longer feed itself, it begins to crumble and fall away. We are exporting many foodstuffs from South America, Mexico and Asia while our own farmers are selling off or losing their land.

For many, the consequence is a decline in health. With large multinational corporations distributing genetically modified grains and grain products throughout the world, we are now seeing the chronic diseases of industrialized nations in third world countries. Obesity is now a worldwide epidemic.

"The prevalence of celiac disease in Middle Eastern and North African countries among low-risk populations is similar to that of Western countries, but is higher in high-risk populations such as those with type 1 diabetes. Clinical presentations in term of gastrointestinal, hematologic, skeletal and liver manifestations are similar between both populations except for a high prevalence of short stature in some Middle Eastern and North African countries." (Division of Gastroenterology, Department of Internal Medicine, American University of Beirut).

In a 2003 study published in the Wake Forest University School of Medicine's *Pediatric Gastroenterology and Nutrition*, a total of 1200 individuals were studied. The conclusion states that "Celiac disease is not rare in the United States and may be as common as in Europe."

A 2004 study from the Maribor General Hospital Department of Pediatrics reported that "The prevalence of celiac disease among first-degree relatives (children) is much higher than the prevalence of the disease in the general population. Most of these patients have an atypical form of the disease and would therefore be overlooked without an active search. Malignancy may be the first manifestation of subclinical (silent) celiac disease."

"Untreated celiac disease increases the risk of over 185 different medical conditions including many chronic brain disorders in adults and children." *(Lancet, April 12, 1997 349: 1096-1097)*

Gluten sensitivity often results in significant serotonin, norepinephrine and dopamine depletion. Gluten sensitivity suppresses gut hormone release adversely affecting cognition, emotions, appetite/satiation and behavior.

Common symptoms include weepiness and irritability, irritable bowel syndrome, autism, depression, ADHD, epilepsy, Down's syndrome, schizophrenia, low IQ children and maternal thyroid disease.

Celiac disease is a severe form of gluten sensitivity. Neurological symptoms include ataxia (balance and gait disorders), seizures, and development of brain lesions and calcifications as well as migraines. Delay in diagnosis and treatment increases the risks of serious harm to the brain and nervous system. *(Braly & Hoggan Dangerous Grains 2003).*

Individuals with celiac disease often experience brain fog in addition to intestinal problems. A new study shows that adhering to a gluten-free diet can lead to improvements in cognition, including increased attention span and improvements in memory.[216]

Up to one-third of all celiac disease patients have been previously diagnosed with IBS and/or lactose intolerance. *(Sanders DS et al. Eur J Gastroenterol Hepatol. 2003;15:407-413).*
Among adults with type 1 diabetes, celiac disease is ten times more prevalent than in the general population. It is very common in children with type 1 diabetes. *(Rotorhead).*

In October 2010 the Department of Neurology, Päijät-Häme Central Hospital in Lahti, Finland, reported on a study involving "381 elderly persons positive for gluten antibodies and confirmed celiac diagnosis. Rheumatoid arthritis and depression were found significantly more often in the subjects with positive tests than control subjects. The significance remained even when known celiac disease cases were excluded."

---

[216] Wiley. "Gluten-free diet relieves 'brain fog' in patients with Celiac disease." ScienceDaily. ScienceDaily, 16 June 2014. <www.sciencedaily.com/releases/2014/06/140616134149.htm>.

Not everyone is gluten sensitive, but research supports an increase in allergies due to GMO grains and foods in as much as 30% of the population.[217, 218]

Going gluten-free for health reasons is not just a fad. When I queried PubMed, I found over 800 journal listings on gluten sensitivity.

Whenever we are told to stop eating certain foods, our visceral response is to resist because we are being asked to deprive ourselves. Our necks stiffen and we dig in our heels, insistent that the problem isn't a food or lifestyle choice.

Eliminating potentially harmful foods like wheat, corn and soy should not be a matter of deprivation and denial; rather, this is an opportunity to embrace traditional and life-building foods, rather than genetically modified and commercialized versions.

Bread and baked goods can be made from alternative grains, and there are many creative ways to go gluten-free. Instead of a sandwich, try slices of cheese with fruit and rice crackers, or steak strips with a side of gluten-free macaroni salad, tabouli or fresh veggies. Snack on hummus and organic non-GMO corn chips. Soups, chilies and stews are always a good choice and many cold soups are very satisfying in the warmer months.

Inspiration Mixes, an Oregon company, offers excellent gluten-free baking mixes. You can enjoy bread, cookies, pie, muffins and pizza without the gluten—and by making them yourself, you save money.

Other Considerations

Beer, wine and fermented drinks have been enjoyed for thousands of years. They were first created to address contaminated water supplies. Unpasteurized versions contain friendly bacteria that aid in digestion. There are many good beers made from rice and sorghum available. Wine and hard liquors are gluten-free.

Body care products include shampoos and cosmetics with wheat germ or other grain-based ingredients. Several companies make GF (gluten-free) products, including Bare Minerals, Enjoy and Jane Iredale. The skin is your largest organ and it can absorb chemicals and contaminates.

---

[217] (Reinagel, 2006)
[218] (Elson M. Haas M. , 2000)

Medications often contain gluten; to obtain the gluten-free version, they must be made on request by a compounding pharmacist. Depression, migraines, skin rashes, chronic pain and erectile dysfunction may result from restricted blood flow due to untreated celiac disease.

When eating at restaurants, try naked sandwiches, sautéed vegetables or a la carte dishes without bread, coatings or pasta. Be bold and ask the manager if the restaurant would consider adding more gluten-free options in the future.

Oats To The Rescue

Oats (*avena sativa*), whether rolled or steel cut, are considered a whole grain because all three parts of the grain are present and preserved during the milling process. The seed portion of the oat plant (known as the groat), rolled, quick-cook, instant, oat flour and oat bran all come from the grass (*Gramineae*) family.

Oats were one of the earliest cultivated grains, believed to have originated in Eurasia and consumed in China before 7000 BC. The ancient Greeks were the first documented people to have made porridge from oats. The English considered oats an inferior grain, while Ireland and Scotland considered it a staple and used the grain in many forms for baking and porridges. It was the British Quakers (thus the name Quaker Oats®) who brought oats to America in the 1600s for cultivation.

Nutrient-packed oats contain vitamin E, B vitamins, calcium, magnesium, potassium, copper, zinc, iron, manganese, phytochemicals, and soluble and insoluble fibers. All of these nutrients in their combined natural state lead to many health benefits.

Oats contain proteins called *avenin* and *gliadin*. Research is showing that non-contaminated oats may be safe for many celiac patients. An article by the Irish gastroenterologist William Dickey in the *European Journal of Gastroenterology and Hepatology* supports the idea that most people with celiac disease can tolerate pure oats, and that only in rare cases do pure oats elicit an adverse reaction. Dickey notes that contamination of commercially viable oats is the cause of most adverse reactions in people with celiac disease.

Researchers know of just three confirmed cases of active celiac disease flaring up in adults after ingesting oats, which indicates that intolerance to oats may be rare.

Clinical monitoring of celiac disease patients who eat oats is still recommended as damage may result even if no symptoms appear.

In January 2011, Cyrex® Labs released a new salivary gluten peptide test proving to be 96% accurate (standard blood tests average only 20% accuracy). This new testing method allows for 19 proteins to be tested instead of four.

A recent study in Spain measured the levels of wheat and barley contamination of oats from Europe, the United States and Canada. Results showed that just 25 of the 134 samples contained no detectable levels of gluten contamination. The other 109 samples all showed wheat, barley and/or rye contamination. The results also showed that contamination levels vary among oats from the same source. *(European Journal of Gastroenterology and Hepatology 20: 492–493; 494–495; 545–554.)*

Why Is Gluten Content Such A Problem?

How gluten affects brain and nerve function is an important consideration for parents of autistic children, MS patients, diabetics and breast cancer patients. If the oats they consume are contaminated with wheat gluten from shared machinery or processing practices, their health could be adversely impacted.

Look for certified gluten-free oats from companies like Bob's Red Mill®. Gluten-free oats may normalize blood pressure, blood sugars, cholesterol and triglycerides, and help with weight management, diabetes, constipation, diarrhea, energy levels and more. Oats can boost testosterone levels by freeing testosterone from its bound state (good for older men with andropause) and help reduce tobacco cravings.

Add a handful of blueberries, cranberries or dried cherries to your oats in the morning. Try using steel cut oats in place of rice or barley in soups and casseroles. The list of options is endless and a new food adventure awaits you.

Fermented Beverages

The earliest consumption of fermented drinks dates back to neolithic African tribesmen who sought out liquid from tree hollows where honey bee hives had been flooded from seasonal rain.

Fermented beers, wines and spirits allowed for a safe and efficient water treatment method, protecting people from E. coli, Giardia and dysentery. The alcohol content of these early beverages was lower than many of today's augmented blends where grain alcohol is used to bring alcohol levels up so that young wines, beers and spirits can be sold sooner.

What If It Isn't Gluten?

It is currently estimated that one-third of Americans are going gluten-free. But what if, for those with non-celiac gluten sensitivity (NCGS), it isn't the gluten that is driving up inflammation markers, but something else? What if it's the nightshade family, or sugar? The reasons why some respond favorably to gluten-free programs while others do not are still not fully understood.

Fructans may be one factor. This group belongs to a diverse family of carbohydrates that are notorious for being difficult to digest. A failure to absorb these compounds into the blood may draw excess water into the digestive tract and agitate its resident bacteria. Wheat proteins known as amylase-trypsin inhibitors stimulate immune cells to release inflammatory cytokines that overexcite the immune system. Wheat is one of the foods that are high in fructans.

Because these carbohydrates are found in many foods—not just grains—a gluten-free or wheat-free diet will not necessarily solve the inflammatory puzzle. One of the types of dietary fiber high in fructans is inulins. Inulin, in its refined form, is found in a wide range of food products including refined wheat flour, sugar and oils.

Inulin is a starchy substance found in a wide variety of fruits, vegetables, grains and herbs, including wheat, rye, barley, spelt, Kamut, brown rice, onions, bananas, leeks, artichoke and asparagus.

The type of inulin that is used for medicine is most commonly obtained by soaking chicory roots in hot water. Inulin is used for high blood fats, including cholesterol and triglycerides, and for weight loss and constipation. It is used as a food additive to improve taste and in gluten-free foods to improve texture.

Could this be why some individuals on a gluten-free diet experience no improvement in symptoms? Researchers are finding a greater number of individuals exhibiting carbohydrate digestion failure; for example, up to 40% of people with Crohn's disease do not absorb carbohydrates properly.

A study released in 2014 reported that intake of sugar-sweetened soda is associated with an increased risk of rheumatoid arthritis (RA) in women. The Centers for

Disease Control and Prevention (CDC) estimate that 1.5 million American adults have RA; 2.5 times more women are affected than men.

The subjects from the Nurses' Health Study (1980-2008) and the Nurses' Health Study II (1991-2009) completed a food frequency questionnaire regarding sugar-sweetened soda consumption (including regular cola, caffeine-free cola and other sugar-sweetened carbonated soda) at the beginning of the study and every four years during the follow-up period. Researchers found that women who consumed one or more servings of sugar-sweetened soda per day had a highly significant (63%) increased risk of developing seropositive RA compared to the women who consumed none or less than one serving per month. When the researchers evaluated the subjects who had onset of RA after age 55, they found that the association was even more significant, with a 164% increased risk of developing seropositive RA.[219]

In natural sources the side effects of fructans may be negated by other components. When we separate out what we believe to be the important "active" ingredients, we leave behind valuable co-factors.

Fructooligosaccharides (FOS) are a form of fructans. They are beneficial for most individuals and are used as an alternative sweetener and probiotic enhancer. They are commonly added to digestive aids called probiotics. The FOS is referred to as a prebiotic because it acts as food for the probiotics, increasing their activity in the large intestine.

Probiotics are commonly called good gut bacteria. They are instrumental in digesting carbohydrates and in B vitamin synthesis in the gut. FOS is between 30 and 50% times sweeter than sugar in commercially prepared syrups. It has been referred to as an essential sugar. When used in commercial foods the amount consumed over the course of a day or week, while safe for those who can properly digest carbohydrates, may be pouring gas on the inflammation fire for those who cannot. Again, more is not always better.

I believe inflammation to be the root cause of chronic illnesses. If you do not digest carbohydrates well, you may need to eliminate wheat and other high-fructan foods and supplement with digestive enzymes. Even if gluten is not the issue, wheat still may be an inflammation trigger.

---

[219] Hu Y, et al. Am J Clin Nutr. 2014 Jul 16. [Epub ahead of print.

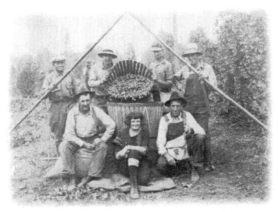

Photo courtesy of Independence Heritage Museum

Most cultures imbibe at least one traditional alcoholic beverage. Often they are reserved for special occasions like baptisms, weddings, bar mitzvahs and funerals. During the holiday season it is common for beer, wine and spirits to be given as gifts.

Early alcoholic beverages contained no herbicides, pesticides or GMO grains; they did, however, sometimes contain high levels of heavy metals. Roman wine contained lead from the piping and cooking vessels.

The following information may illustrate why it has been so difficult for 75% of my clients to give up the occasional beer or nightly glass of wine.

Beer

Late Stone Age beer jugs found by an archaeologist established that deliberately fermented beverages existed at least as early as 10,000 BC. It has been suggested that beer may have preceded bread as a dietary staple. The invention of bread and beer has been heralded as vital to the development of civilization.

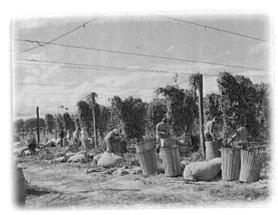

Practically all hops in the U.S. are Grown in the Willamette Valley of Oregon Photo Courtesy of Independence Heritage Museum.

In every culture, from hunter-gatherers to nation-states, alcoholic beverages are often an important part of social events. Drinking often plays a significant role in social interaction—some believe mainly because of alcohol's neurological effects.

Fermentation is the process whereby microorganisms are utilized to produce alcoholic beverages such as wine, beer and cider. Fermentation is also employed in the leavening of bread, for preservation, and to create lactic acid in sour foods such as sauerkraut, dry sausages, kimchi, pickles (vinegar) and yogurt. Fermented foods protect and maintain healthy bacteria in the digestive tract. Fermentation was a key preservation tool prior to refrigeration and canning, and in areas where ice is not available.

Beer is one of the world's oldest prepared beverages, possibly dating back to the early Neolithic or 9500 BC when cereal was first farmed, as recorded in the written history of ancient Egypt and Mesopotamia.

The earliest known chemical evidence of beer dates to circa 3500–3100 BC and comes from the site of Godin Tepe in the Zagros Mountains of western Iran. A prayer to the goddess Ninkasi, known as The Hymn to Ninkasi, served as both a prayer and a method of remembering the recipe for beer in a culture with few literate people. The Ebla tablets, discovered in 1974 in Syria and dating back to 2500 BC, reveal that the city produced a range of beers including one named Ebla, after the city. A beer made from rice, which, unlike sake, was prepared for fermentation by malting, was made in China around 7000 BC.

The thegreatestbeers.com reports " Beer was spread through Europe by Germanic and Celtic tribes as far back as 3000 BC, and it was mainly brewed on a domestic scale. The product that the early Europeans drank might not be recognized as beer by most people today. Alongside the basic starch source, the early European beers might contain fruits, honey, numerous types of plants, spices and other substances such as narcotic herbs. What they did not contain was hops, as that was a later addition first mentioned in Europe around 822 by a Carolingian Abbot and again in 1067 by Abbess Hildegard of Bingen."[220]

In 1516, William IV, Duke of Bavaria, adopted the *Reinheitsgebot* (purity law), perhaps the oldest food quality regulation still in use. According to this law, the only allowed ingredients in beer are water, hops and barley malt. Beer produced before the Industrial Revolution continued to be made and sold on a domestic scale, although by the 7th century AD, beer was also being produced and sold by European

---

[220] This section similar to here: http://www.thegreatestbeers.com/katcef/beer-101/history-of-beer/

monasteries. During the Industrial Revolution, the production of beer moved from artisanal manufacture to industrial manufacture, and domestic manufacture ceased by the end of the 19th century.

Today, the brewing industry is a global business, consisting of several dominant multinational companies and many thousands of smaller producers ranging from brewpubs to regional breweries. The Pacific Northwest is famous for its microbrews and has received national and international recognition for the specialty beers. In 2006 more than 133 billion liters (35 billion gallons) of beer were sold, earning total global revenues of $294.5 billion.

Health Effects

The moderate consumption of alcohol (4 oz of spirits, 6-8 oz of beer and wine) is associated with a decreased risk of cardiac disease, stroke and cognitive decline. The long-term effects of alcohol abuse, however, include the risk of developing alcoholism and alcoholic liver disease. Anyone with elevated liver enzymes or hepatitis C should avoid all alcohol.

Brewer's yeast is a rich source of nutrients used in the fermentation of beer. Beer can contain significant amounts of nutrients, including magnesium, selenium, potassium, phosphorus, biotin and B vitamins. Beer is sometimes referred to as "liquid bread". Filtered beer may contain less nutrients.

A 2005 Japanese study found that low-alcohol beer may possess strong anti-cancer properties. Another study found that non-alcoholic beer provides the cardiovascular benefits associated with moderate consumption of alcoholic beverages. However, other research suggests that the primary health benefits derived from alcoholic beverages is due to the alcohol.

The key, of course, is moderation. Beer can be calorie-dense and estrogenic, so watch out for the dreaded "beer belly".

AppleJack

When the Romans arrived in England in 55 BC, they were reported to have found the local Kentish villagers drinking a delicious cider-like beverage made from apples. According to ancient records, the Romans and their leader, Julius Caesar, embraced the pleasant pursuit with enthusiasm. How long the locals had been making this apple drink prior to the arrival of the Romans is a mystery. By the beginning of the 9th century, cider drinking was well established in Europe.

Historical information found on drinkfocus.com reports "After the Norman Conquest of 1066, cider consumption became widespread in England and orchards were established specifically to produce cider apples. During medieval times, cider making was an important industry. Monasteries sold vast quantities of their strong, spiced cider to the public. Farm laborers received a cider allowance as part of their wages, and the amount increased during haymaking. English cider making probably peaked around the mid 17th century, when almost every farm had its own cider orchard and press."

Early English settlers introduced cider to America by bringing with them seeds for cultivating cider apples. During the colonial period, grains did not thrive well and were costly to import. On the other hand, apple orchards were plentiful, making apples cheap and readily obtainable. Alcoholic beverages were forbidden by the early American Puritans, however, apple cider was not prohibited as it was made from fruit and not grain. Safer than water and easier and cheaper to produce than beer or wine, cider was typically the first drink of the day.

In the Colonial period and up to the middle of the 19th century, cider just meant fermented apple juice. During that time, it was the most popular and important beverage in America. Consumption of cider increased steadily during the eighteenth century, due in part to the efforts of the legendary Johnny Appleseed, who planted many apple trees in the Midwest. Cider regained popularity during the 20th century, but demand was largely for the mass-produced variety. Only in recent years has traditional cider making finally triumphed.

Water Of Life

The Gaelic *usquebaugh*, meaning "Water of Life", phonetically became "usky" and then "whiskey" in English. Scotland has internationally protected the term "Scotch"; to be labeled as Scotch it must be produced in Scotland.

"Eight bolls of malt to Friar John Cor wherewith to make aqua vitae." This entry appeared in the Exchequer Rolls in 1494 and seems to be the earliest documented record of distilling in Scotland.

"Scotland's great Renaissance king, James IV (1488-1513) was fond of "ardent spirits". When the king visited Dundee in 1506, a payment to the local barber for a supply of aqua vitae for the king's pleasure was recorded. In 1505, the Guild of Barber Surgeons in Edinburgh was granted a monopoly over the manufacture of aqua vitae—a fact that reflects the spirit's perceived medicinal properties as well as the medicinal talents of the barbers." (whiskyman.com)

In early 2010 three crates of Mackinlay's Rare Old Highland Malt Whiskey were found under the floor of John Shackleton's 1908 Nimrod expedition shelter in Antarctica. The original recipe for this particular breed of Scotch has been lost and master blenders the world over are waiting with great anticipation for the opportunity to take a sniff of this Scotch. Authorities in New Zealand's Antarctic Museum in Christchurch plan to extract small samples for analysis and then the bottles will be returned to Antarctica for posterity.

Legend says St. Patrick introduced distilling to Ireland in the 5th century, and it is believed Patrick acquired the knowledge in Spain and France. The distilling process was initially applied to perfume, then to wine, and finally adapted to fermented mashes of cereals in countries where grapes were not plentiful.

The spirit was universally termed aqua vitae ("water of life") and was commonly made in monasteries. It was chiefly used for medicinal purposes, being prescribed for the preservation of health, the prolongation of life, and for the relief of colic, palsy and even smallpox.

The art of distilling is believed to have been brought to Europe by Irish missionary monks. The secrets also traveled with the Dalriadic Scots when they arrived in Kintyre Scotland around 500 AD. The knowledge of distilling spread through monastery communities. The oldest licensed whiskey distillery in the world, Bushmills, lies in Northern Ireland and received its license by Jacob VI in 1608.

Sine Metu, meaning "without fear", appears on every bottle of Jameson whiskey. This has been Jameson's motto since the founding of the Dublin Distillery in 1780. John Jameson set new standards for the distillation of whiskey. Discovering that certain strains of barley made better whiskey than others, he persuaded local farmers to grow the desired grains by providing them with seed each spring. By 1820, John Jameson & Sons had become the second largest distilling company in Ireland.

A Tot If You Please

Rum was not commonly available until after 1650, when it was imported from the Caribbean. The cost of rum dropped after the colonists began importing molasses and cane sugar and began distilling it themselves. By 1657, a rum distillery was operating in Boston. It was highly successful and within a generation, the production of rum became colonial New England's largest and most prosperous industry. Almost every important town, from Massachusetts to the Carolinas, had a rum distillery to meet the local demand, which had increased dramatically. Rum was often enjoyed in mixed drinks, including flip. This was a favorite winter beverage made of rum and beer sweetened with sugar and warmed by plunging a red-hot fireplace poker into the serving mug.

Shaken, Not Stirred

It was also during the 17th century that Franciscus Sylvius (or Franz de la Boe), a professor of medicine at the University of Leyden, distilled spirits from grain. This spirit was generally flavored with juniper berries. The resulting beverage was known as *junever*, the Dutch word for juniper. The French changed the name to *genievre*, which the English changed to "geneva" and then modified to "gin".

Originally used for medicinal purposes, gin was not often consumed socially. However in 1690, England passed "An Act for the Encouraging of the Distillation of Brandy and Spirits from Corn" and within four years the annual production of spirits, mostly gin, reached nearly one million gallons.

South Of The Border

Tequila is distilled from the sap of the agave plant indigenous to Mexico, not the mescal cactus, as many people believe. This clear peppery liquor was traditionally used as a dietary aid, consumed following a heavy meal to stimulate digestion. Many people still drink tequila along with rich Tex-Mexican food, loaded with fat and cheese. The Jaime family in Arandes, Jalisco, Mexico has been growing "all natural" Weber Blue Agave for the tequila industry for over 100 years. No pesticides, chemical weed control, hormonal fertilizers or chemicals are used to grow or speed the distillation process of Oregon's only family owned tequila.

If you like to drink alcoholic beverages, make sure they come from reputable distilleries and are made from pure ingredients. Ask if the beverage contains grain alcohol; if it is, try one made with grain less likely to be a GMO product or contaminated with herbicides.

Protestant leaders such as Luther and Calvin, the Anglican Church and even the Puritans did not differ substantially from the teachings of the Catholic Church when it came to alcohol. They believed alcohol was a gift of God and created to be used in moderation for pleasure, enjoyment and health; drunkenness was regarded as a sin.

Wine, Ruby in Color

Wine is the second most (or possibly the most) oldest of the fermented beverages developed. According to an ancient Persian fable, wine was the accidental discovery of a princess seeking to end her life with what she thought was poison. Instead, she experienced the elixir's intoxicating effects and it released her from the anxieties of royal court life.

Experts agree wine probably dates to 6000 BC Mesopotamia, where wild grape vines grew. The drink was savored by royalty and priests, while commoners drank beer, mead and ale. The ancient Egyptians were the first culture to document the process of wine-making.

Wine-making made its way to Greece, where it permeated all aspects of society: literature, mythology, medicine, leisure and religion. The Romans took vine clippings from Greece back to Italy, and centers of viticulture soon developed in France, Germany, Italy, Spain, Portugal and the rest of Europe.[221]

---

[221] http://www.winepros.org/wine101/history.htm

From the Bible to ancient legends, tales of intoxication by ingesting fermented grapes abound. In addition, fossilized vines add proof to the fact that the earliest humans recognized the pleasures of this tantalizing liquid.

> *"Good wine is a necessity of life for me."*
> – Thomas Jefferson

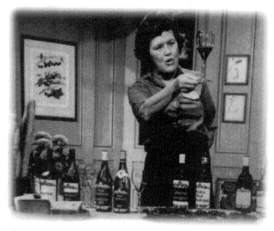

"Wine is a living liquid containing no preservatives. Its life cycle comprises youth, maturity, old age and death.
When not treated with reasonable respect it will sicken and die." – Julia Child

From Honey To Happy Mead

The history of mead dates back 20,000 to 40,000 years and originates on the African continent. In Africa during the dry season, wild bees would nest in tree hollows, and during the wet season the hollows would fill with water. Water, honey, osmotolerant yeast, time and *voila*—mead is born. As successive waves of people left Africa they took with them some knowledge of mead and mead-making. Not until the time of Louis Pasteur, in the mid-1800s, did man become aware of yeast as the life form responsible for fermentation.

Honey was prized throughout history; it was often available only to royalty and with time the tradition of mead was only sustained in the monasteries of Europe.[222, 223]

Eventually mead-making spread throughout Europe, India and China. But mead-making died out as people became urbanized. However, mead has resurged in popularity in the 21st century, and individuals are once more making traditional mead as well as flavor-blended vintages.

In medieval times Christmas was quite a pagan celebration. Foods were heavily spiced if the lord of the manor was wealthy enough to purchase clove, cardamom, cinnamon and ginger from travelers and tradesmen. The lady of the manor would combine these herbs with meats as a preservative and with wine or mead to improve digestion and prevent food poisoning.

A-Wassailing We Go

The text of the carol employs noun and verb forms of "wassail", a word derived from the Old Norse *ves heil* and the Old English *was hál* meaning "be in good health" or "be fortunate". The phrase found first use as a simple greeting, but the Danish-speaking inhabitants of England seem to have turned *was hail,* and the reply *drink hail,* into a drinking formula adopted widely by the population of England— the Norman conquerors who arrived in the 11th century regarded the toast as distinctive of the English natives.

"Wassail" appears in English literature as a salute as early as the 8th century epic *Beowulf,* in references such as "warriors' wassail and words of power."[224]

Wassail Recipe [225]

Makes approx. 4 quarts

Ingredients
4 cups freshly pressed apple cider
1 cups orange juice
1 cups cranberry juice
2 pints heavy winter ale*

[222] Levi-Strauss C.: From honey to ashes (1966)
[223] Enright M. J.: Lady with a mead cup, Four courts press (1996)
[224] http://www.history.org/Almanack/life/Christmas/hist_wassail.cfm
[225] http://www.history.uk.com/recipes/traditional-wassail-recipes/

3 cups port*
4 small tart/sweet apples, peeled and cored
1 lemon
1 lime
1 orange
1 tsp ground cardamom
3 small or 1.5 large cinnamon sticks
15 whole cloves
6 whole allspice
1 tsp grated fresh ginger
4 Tbsp brown sugar
1 Tbsp cold butter

*2 pints sherry or Madeira wine and 1cup rum are often substituted for ale and port, resulting in a sweeter flavor and lighter body.

Pre-heat oven to 350 degrees. Pack 1 tbsp. of brown sugar and ¼ tbsp. of butter into the core of each apple. Place apples in a small baking dish and fill the dish with ½ inch of water (to keep apples from burning or sticking to the bottom).

When oven is preheated, bake apples uncovered for 45 min. to one hour or until tender and soft, but not mushy. Drain the water. Quarter each baked apple (or divide into eighths depending on the number of guests).

Combine cardamom, cloves, allspice and ginger in a small piece of cheesecloth, and tie closed with twine to form a spice packet.

In a large stockpot or slow cooker combine apple cider, cranberry juice, orange juice, (plus ale, port/rum, wine as desired), and the juice of one lemon and one lime.

Place cinnamon directly into liquids and stir to infuse. Submerge spice packet in stockpot. Stir apples into stockpot (they'll ultimately float on top and begin to soften, fall apart and add a creamy quality to the liquid).

Simmer on medium/high (never boiling) for two hours until hot spices are thoroughly infused and apples have begun to dissolve. Remove spice packet and pour into "wassail bowl" if not using stockpot or slow cooker. Be prepared to reheat until the wassail bowl is empty.

Garnish the wassail bowl by floating thin slices of the remaining lemon, limes and oranges on top.

Serve in small mugs with a sizable piece of apple in each mug.

Osteoporosis is a skeletal condition characterized by a decrease in overall bone density. It affects elderly individuals around the world, particularly postmenopausal women. The disorder often goes unnoticed until a fracture occurs as a result of brittle bones (not thinner, flexible bones). [226]

There have been several studies of long-lived individuals around the world that show that diet and exercise are key to maintaining healthy bones. Movement and sunshine, not medication, will help prevent brittle bones.

In the past, researchers thought low estrogen caused osteoporosis. This was because most of the patients were post-menopausal women, and because estrogen does influence the bone-forming activity of osteoblasts. However, further research has found that a decline in estrogen levels is not a major cause of osteoporosis. Researchers have also learned that menopause is not a period of estrogen decline but rather a time of progesterone decline. [227, 228]

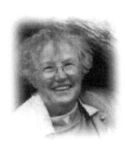

Another theory held that calcium deficiency caused osteoporosis, but per capita Americans consume more dairy than any other society and also have the highest occurrences of osteoporosis. We learned that patients were being given too much calcium and neglecting not only vitamin D, which is critical to bone health, but also a host of other minerals necessary for healthy bone formation.

Older people have lower levels of vitamin D. Their digestive systems do not absorb nutrients well, especially minerals, due to low levels of hydrochloric acid which is necessary to dissolve minerals. Hyperparathyroidism is another factor linked with osteoporosis incidence. The cumulative effects of inactivity, impaired parathyroid function and vitamin and mineral deficiencies over the years lead to osteoporosis. [229, 230]

---

[226] (Tabers, 2001)
[227] (Pamela Wartian Smith, HRT: The Answers, 2003)
[228] (Kenna Stephenson, 2004)
[229] (Carl Germano, 1999)
[230] (Susan E. Brown, 2000)

Walnuts are rich in alpha-linolenic acid, an omega-3 fatty acid that helps decrease the rate of bone breakdown and keeps bone formation constant, according to a 2007 *Nutrition Journal* study. Brazil nuts are also great sources of magnesium. Eat raw nuts and seeds daily to boost bone health.

Oysters: The oyster is the best source of zinc, a mineral important for immune function, growth, taste, smell, wound healing and dozens of enzymatic reactions in the body.

Leafy Greens: Salads and steamed greens are packed with bone-building nutrients, particularly calcium, magnesium and vitamin K. Vitamin K is critical in forming bone proteins and cuts calcium loss in urine. Research shows too little of this fat-soluble vitamin increases the risk of hip fractures.

Beans*: Beans, especially pinto, black, white and kidney, provide a good boost of magnesium and some calcium. The U.S. Dietary Guidelines for Americans recommends at least 2.5 cups of beans and other legumes (peas, lentils) weekly.

Fish: We need vitamin D so our bodies can absorb calcium. Vitamin D deficiency, in addition to vitamin K deficiency, is linked to hip fracture. In fact, 50% of women with osteoporosis who were hospitalized for hip fracture had signs of vitamin D deficiency, according to a scientific review by the American Medical Association. The best fish is Alaskan salmon. A small serving of salmon—only 3.5 ounces— gives you 90% of the daily recommended amount of vitamin D (it is a good idea to get your vitamin D levels tested and take supplemental vitamin D3 daily if you have osteoporosis).

Exercising & Osteoporosis

You might think the friction of exercise would lead to fractures. In fact, using your muscles helps protect your bones. According to the Mayo Clinic, "Starting an exercise program can help you avoid falls—and may keep your bones from getting weaker. For postmenopausal women, regular physical activity can increase muscle strength, improve balance, make you better able to carry out daily tasks and activities, maintain or improve your posture, relieve or decrease pain and improve your sense of well-being." [231, 232, 233]

---

[231] (Susan Brown, 2000)
[232] (Jensen, 1986)

A new syndrome called "osteosarcopenic obesity" that links the deterioration of bone density and muscle mass with obesity has been identified by researchers. The syndrome explains how many obese individuals experience a triad of problems that place them at a higher risk of falling and breaking bones. Researchers note that the work stands to remind people to consider the damage that can be done to all parts of the body if they are overweight.[234]

Spending too much time in front of the TV or computer can lead to weight gain, stress and heart disease. The shift to a more sedentary lifestyle has also been bad for our bones. A pair of papers published in the *Proceedings of the National Academy of Sciences* suggests that humans evolved lighter joint bones relatively recently in our evolutionary history as a response to changes in physical activity. "The lightly-built skeleton of modern humans has a direct and important impact on bone strength and stiffness," says Tim Ryan, an anthropologist at Penn State University and a co-author on the second study. That's because lightness can translate to weakness—more broken bones and a higher incidence of osteoporosis and age-related bone loss.

Previous studies suggested walking upright put more pressure on joints, which made them longer and leaner; others argued that a decrease in physical activity or changes in diet were linked to these skeletal changes.

Recently, scientists have zeroed in on trabecular bone, the sponge-like material found at the ends of the bones that form joints. Modern humans have lower trabecular bone density within specific bones than their ancestors who lived as hunter-gatherers.[235]

Current studies show that inactive elderly women with osteoporosis can regain 15% bone mass by engaging in mild weight-lifting exercise three days per week. Bone support medications have an efficacy of 6%.

Exercises to Build Bone Strength

Strength training exercises, especially those for the back: Strength training includes the use of free weights, weight machines, resistance bands or water exercises to strengthen the muscles and bones in your arms and upper spine. Strength training can also work directly on your bones to slow mineral loss.

---

[233] (Colbin, 1998)
[234] Florida State University. "Obesity can amplify bone, muscle loss." ScienceDaily. ScienceDaily, 16 April 2014. <www.sciencedaily.com/releases/2014/04/140416162452.htm>.
[235] http://www.smithsonianmag.com/science -nature/switching -farming -made-human-joint-bones-lighter -180953711/

Weight-bearing aerobic activities: Weight-bearing aerobic activities involve doing aerobic exercise on your feet, with your bones supporting your weight. Examples include walking, dancing, low-impact aerobics, elliptical training machines, stair climbing and gardening. These types of exercise work directly on the bones in your legs, hips and lower spine to slow mineral loss.

Flexibility exercises: Being able to move your joints through their full range of motion helps you maintain good balance and prevent muscle injury. Increased flexibility can also help improve your posture. When your joints are stiff, abdominal and chest muscles become tight, pulling you forward and giving you a stooped posture.

Stability and balance exercises: "Fall prevention is important for people who have osteoporosis. Stability and balance exercises help your muscles work together in a way that helps keep you more stable and less likely to fall. Simple exercises such as standing on one leg or movement-based exercises such as tai chi can improve your stability and balance. "*(Atlantis Physical Therapy)*

Exercises that Exacerbate Osteoporosis

If you have osteoporosis, don't do high-impact exercises such as jumping, running or jogging. These activities increase compression in your spine and lower extremities and can lead to fractures in weakened bones. Choose exercises with slow, controlled movements.

Also, avoid exercises in which you bend forward and twist your waist, such as touching your toes or doing sit-ups. These movements put pressure on the bones in your spine, increasing your risk of compression fractures. Other activities that may require you to bend or twist forcefully at the waist are golf, tennis, bowling and some yoga poses.

So get out and get moving—and drag a friend, dog or loved one along with you!

Osteoarthritis & Zinc

Osteoarthritis, especially in the knee, is a fairly common condition and a leading cause of disability. Other afflicted areas can include the shoulder or hips. Characterized by the destruction of cartilage tissue in joints, there is a lack of effective therapies because the underlying molecular causes have been unclear. A study published on February 13, 2014 in the journal *Cell* reveals osteoarthritis-related tissue damage is caused by a molecular pathway that is involved in regulating and responding to zinc levels inside of cartilage cells.

When the cartilage breaks down, the bones rub together, causing pain, swelling and stiffness. This tissue destruction is caused by proteins called matrix-degrading enzymes which are produced by cartilage cells. The enzymes degrade the extracellular matrix, the structural support system that surrounds cells and holds them together. Because matrix-degrading enzymes require zinc to function, zinc levels inside of cartilage cells may play a role in osteoarthritis.

What Is Zinc Beneficial For?

- Zinc may stimulate the formation of bones; impaired bone growth in adolescents may occur as a result of (even minor) zinc deficiency.
- Fibromyalgia patients are often found to have low zinc levels. Lower zinc levels in fibromyalgia patients is associated with a greater number of tender points.
- Zinc facilitates the healing of fractures.
- Night muscle cramps may occur as a result of zinc deficiency.
- Zinc may improve muscle strength.
- Osteoporosis patients are often found to have low serum and bone zinc levels.
- Zinc may alleviate the symptoms of psoriatic and rheumatoid arthritis. Clinical studies have shown supplemental zinc may alleviate the joint swelling and morning stiffness associated with rheumatoid arthritis.
- Zinc may alleviate scleroderma.
- White specks on the fingernails or nails that split easily may occur as a result of zinc deficiency.

What are the downsides to this mineral?

1. Zinc competes with copper and iron for the same receptor sites and may reduce magnesium along with other minerals. It is best if this mineral is taken separately from other mineral supplements.
2. Zinc may inhibit the absorption of tetracyclines.
3. Excessive zinc intake may cause anemia.
4. Excessive zinc intake may contribute to atherosclerosis.
5. Large doses of zinc (over 150 mg per day) may reduce the body's production of HDL cholesterol. However, optimal zinc levels may enhance the production of HDL cholesterol.

How Much Is Safe To Take?

The optimal daily allowance (ODA) of zinc (for adults) is 15-50 mg per day. The recommended therapeutic dosage of supplemental zinc for athletes is 30-60 mg zinc per day.

For the common cold, try an initial dose of 50 mg of zinc followed by 25 mg every two hours (using zinc lozenges or zinc tablets slowly dissolved in the mouth, but not rapidly swallowed). The form of zinc should be zinc acetate or zinc gluconate.

The best food sources of zinc are oysters, beef, lamb and liver. Unfortunately, the mineral zinc is tightly bound by phytic acid in plant foods making it hard to gain adequate amounts to correct deficiencies.

My suggestion is to supplement with about 30 mg of good quality zinc from a reliable practitioner, and incorporate zinc-rich foods in your diet.

Why Is It So Hard To Feed Our Elders?

In the United States, one in twelve seniors does not have access to adequate food due to lack of money or other financial resources.

I have several clients who often have to decide between forgoing medication, transportation or food. If they are living with dietary restrictions and have a pet, the situation may be dire.

These individuals are the victims of time, age and false promises. Some of them are like an acquaintance whose spouse was the primary income holder; when he passed away, so did the retirement income, leaving her with only her social security. Yes, this may be the result of poor planning, but how many reading this can throw stones?

I'm not one who believes in living on the dole, but when I hear of elderly women losing their food stamps or having their HUD housing allowance cut because they earned a little extra money at the spring fair or for working a part-time temp job, I get annoyed. One eighty-two-year-old client has to provide itemized lists of medications and nutrients each month to justfify her food assistance; she has a medical file three inches thick.

In the Pacific Northwest we are blessed with a climate that allows for agricultural abundance. As a child, my mother, aunt and others in the area began planning the garden in January. By August, jars were filling the shelves with jam, fruit and vegetables. Later, when we got our first big freezer, it was filled with meat, fish and other foods. We knew how to be self-sufficient, as did many of today's elderly. But they no longer have the health or resources to plant a garden on their own anymore.

Recent research at the University of Illinois, using data from the National Health and Nutrition Examination Survey (NHANES), revealed that the seniors who are dealing with hunger are also facing negative health and nutrition outcomes.

"In 2011, 8.35 percent of Americans over age 60 faced the threat of hunger—that translates to 4.8 million people," said Craig Gundersen, University of Illinois professor in agricultural strategy in the Department of Agricultural and Consumer Economics and executive director of the National Soybean Research Laboratory, who led the data analysis on the study.

A decreased intake of calories, vitamins and other nutrients puts this demographic at risk for a wide variety of ailments. Common issues include falls, dehydration, dementia, fractures, diabetes and heart disease. With adequate nutrient intake, these individuals can maintain their independence, health and productivity without prescription medications or repeat doctor visits.

The Federation of American Societies for Experimental Biology (FASEB) reported that lower dietary consumption of EPA and DHA, the active components of high quality fish oil, might be risk factors for cognitive decline. There is growing evidence that very long chain omega-3 fatty acids are beneficial for maintaining cognitive, heart, nerve and general health. "Intake of fatty fish such as salmon, tuna and trout can help prevent cognitive decline; our preliminary data support previous research showing intake of these types of fish have health benefits," one researcher said.

Community gardens allow people to connect, socialize and feed one another by working together. There is so much that can be done without involving the federal or state governments. It is time for communities to take back control of their health.

Potassium: Do You Need It?

I have a growing number of elderly clients on low-salt diets who are taking potassium supplements. This concerns me because of the delicate biological balance between these two minerals. When I ask clients about the foods they are eating to replace potassium, the answer is often bananas. This can be a problematic food for diabetics if they are not consuming adequate amounts of other fruits and vegetables to maintain healthy blood sugars and mineral balance.

Potassium is necessary for proper functioning of the heart, kidneys and other organs. It works in conjunction with sodium in the body. This mineral is easily obtainable from a diet rich with fruits, vegetables and whole foods.

Many Americans do not eat a healthy diet, especially the elderly or chronically ill, and may be deficient in potassium. Low potassium is associated with a risk of high blood pressure, heart disease, stroke, arthritis, cancer, digestive disorders and infertility. For this condition, doctors will simply recommend potassium supplements and bananas—which drives me, well, bananas.

Potassium Deficiencies Are More Common In People Who:

1. Use diuretics and birth control pills
2. Have physically demanding jobs
3. Are high-performance athletes
4. Have celiac, ulcerative colitis, IBS or Crohn's disease
5. Have an eating disorder
6. Smoke
7. Abuse alcohol or drugs

The Institute of Medicine recommends 4700 mg of potassium for the average adult. This number is different for endurance athletes, firefighters, marathon runners, and pregnant and breastfeeding women. These individuals need to carefully monitor their potassium and salt intake to prevent a condition known as hyponatremia.

Hyponatremia is an electrolyte disturbance in which the sodium ion concentration in the plasma is lower than normal. Normal serum sodium levels are between approximately 135 and 145 mEq/L (135-145 mmol/L). Hyponatremia is generally defined as a serum level of less than 135 mEq/L and is considered severe when the serum level is below 125 mEq/L.

Many conditions including congestive heart failure, liver failure, kidney failure and pneumonia have an associated risk of hyponatremia. It can also be caused by drinking too much water (polydipsia).

Balance Is Critical

Many healthcare providers will tell you this is not a common occurrence, but I routinely see elderly clients with dehydration. Some have ended up in the hospital for emergency rehydration. Many also have health conditions where supplemental potassium is contraindicated, such as kidney disease and congestive heart disease. All had low-to-normal sodium levels before the hospitalization and several were told to take potassium supplements. Additionally, the clients or their family members often express concerns over loss of memory or cognitive function. Confusion is a common symptom of dehydration and poor electrolyte balance.

Let's take a look at healthy foods that will help maintain your electrolyte balance without the risk of overdosing on potassium or elevating your blood sugars.

Natural Food Sources Of Potassium Include:

Mung Beans
Kelp/dulse
Molasses
Avocados
Almonds
Pistachios
Cashews
Peanuts
Black and green tea
Parsley
Watercress
Spinach
Kale
Chard
Beet greens
Broccoli
Tomato paste
Potatoes
Flounder
Cod (canned)
Salmon

Sardines
Figs (high glycemic)
Raisins (high glycemic)
Dates (high glycemic)
Bananas (high glycemic)

The FDA has determined that foods containing at least 350 milligrams of potassium can have the following label: "Diets containing foods that are good sources of potassium and low in sodium may reduce the risk of high blood pressure and stroke."

What Are The Risks Of Taking Potassium?

Side effects: Upset stomach. Some people have allergies to potassium supplements.

Interactions: Potassium supplements may not be safe if you take certain medicines for diabetes, high blood pressure or heart disease.

Warnings: People with kidney disease, diabetes, heart disease, Addison's disease, stomach ulcers or other health problems should never take potassium supplements without talking to a doctor first.

Overdose: Signs of a potassium overdose include confusion, tingling sensation in the limbs, low blood pressure, irregular heartbeat, weakness and coma. Get emergency medical help immediately.

Healthy travel snack suggestions:

- **Trail mix.** I use raw nuts as they are healthier and less likely to cause GI upset than roasted, which can contain damaged oils. I combine the mixed nuts with dried blueberries, cranberries, cherries and dark chocolate chips. This blend provides antioxidants, essential fats, protein and minerals.
- **Veggie sticks.** I use sliced fennel bulb (helps prevent gas), snap peas, carrots, celery, red bell peppers and raw yam,.
- **Sliced apples, pears and pineapple.** The pineapple helps keep the apples and pears from browning.
- **Finger steaks.** Before leaving I make marinated finger strips of well-done elk, beef or chicken. I only make enough for lunch so I'm not letting it sit around all day. Make sure the meat is chilled thoroughly or even frozen before tucking it into your carry-on.
- **Water.** Keeping yourself well-hydrated can help prevent you from catching a virus, so prevalent on planes and in airports. I carry a container of Airborne® with me and load one or more water bottles with it to help support my immune system. These types of products also contain vitamin C and B vitamins for energy.
- **Meal replacement bars and nut bars like Kind Plus®.** These are handy for breakfast or snacks while sightseeing, and require no refrigeration.
- **Hand sanitizer.** I prefer the ones made with peppermint oil and ethanol, such as EO® hand sanitizing spray.

After arriving at your destination, follow these guidelines:

- Eat a breakfast that contains protein and complex carbohydrates like oatmeal, nuts and fruit.
- Have at least one glass of warm water with fresh lemon squeezed into it and the pulp and rind added. This will activate the liver and bowels.
- Minimize dairy as it can be mucus-forming and lead to chest/nasal/gut congestion and constipation.
- Keep bowels moving with a regular fiber supplement; I recommend plain psyllium seed. Start with one-fourth the amount listed on the label and over two weeks slowly increase to the amount listed on the label.
- Make lunch your biggest meal.
- Begin each meal with a salad and use vinegar as the dressing on the salad or on steamed vegetables. By adding as little as a tablespoon of vinegar to a

meal you can lower the overall glycemic load, reduce blood sugar and blood pressure and stimulate healthy digestion, reducing the likelihood of GERD or heartburn.

- Make dinner your smallest meal and load up on vegetables. You will rest better and have more energy for the next day of sightseeing.
- Go easy on the coffee as it can increase muscle cramps and lower back pain if kidneys are overworked.
- Keep alcohol, fried foods and desserts to a minimum. All of these can elevate blood sugars, which can make you feel fatigued the next day.
- Get out and move every day.
- Drink plenty of water: 4-8 glasses a day of 6 to 8 ounces will prevent water retention, light-headedness, headaches and low back pain. Tip: drink in small sips, this keeps you from running to every bathroom in town.

Eating healthy while traveling can prevent unwanted weight gain, jet lag and water retention while keeping energy levels up.

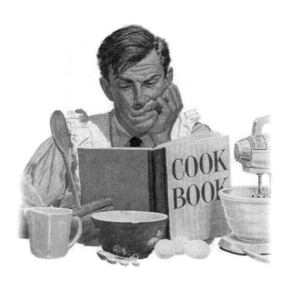

Building your health starts with resolving to take responsibility and to be proactive.

Build Your Team

I hope you enjoy a great relationship with your medical provider. If you don't, you should think about why that is and what you are willing to do about it. You are paying for a service—customer service, respect and cooperation should be expected.

Your health is like an old-fashioned wagon wheel: you are the inner hub and your health is the outer rim, and each of the spokes that support you are your healthcare providers. They are a collection of individuals and modalities that help you stay well. They should be willing to work together and respect the others' roles; no single spoke can hold the wheel together.

This team can include family nurse practitioners, compounding pharmacists, massage therapists, chiropractors, acupuncturists, herbalists, biofeedback specialists, oosteopaths, environmental dentists, ophthalmologists and nutritionists.

Being Proactive

Retirees are often preyed upon by the health industry. They are subjected to sales pitches for everything from erectile dysfunction to age spots. Please be aware of this and get a second opinion before buying the latest panacea promising instant health.

My clients often come in with bags and boxes of supplements. Most of them are outdated, poor quality and redundant. More is not always better and it is important to be just as careful about what supplements you take as you are about prescription medications.

If you need assistance in choosing supplements, ask a pharmacist, medical practitioner or natural healthcare provider who has training in nutritional therapy. Don't simply take the advice of a sales representative, unless you know they can be trusted.

When it comes to nutraceuticals, keep it simple, high quality and food-based. Vitamin and mineral synthetics are not ideal; neither are products loaded with chemical additives like propylene glycol (food-grade antifreeze). As much as I like

Costco®, I do not recommend the majority of their supplements because of the "other ingredients" list containing artificial colors, flavors, chemicals, fillers, binders, preservatives and who knows what else.

Eat real food; I can't stress this enough. With costs increasing due to inflation and fuel taxes, it is even more worthwhile to cut out processed foods. Additives, flavorings, glitzy packages and questionable health claims falsely lure you into purchasing synthetic foods that are bad for your wallet and your health.

Instead, choose fresh and organic, preferably from local farmers. Cook extra and keep leftovers in the refrigerator and freezer. If the consumer's food budget goes to mega-corporations, it does nothing to help local agriculture and our community.

Keep copies of your medical records. Recently I had a medical practitioner tell me they had to close the office doors for a day due to power outages; it wasn't due to lighting but because they could not access the patients' medical records that are now commonly stored on Internet cloud servers. By having a hard copy of your records you know when they have been altered and can have them available for copying when changing providers or seeing specialists. These records are yours; you have paid for them and you have a right and responsibility to see them. This ensures that medications, histories and personal information are accurate.

Grow a garden, even if it is only a container garden of fresh herbs. This helps lower costs and allows you to take control of your food supply. It also helps to be in touch with Mother Nature. My husband told me that when working with explosives, the handlers reach down and touch the soil to discharge accumulated static charge built up from clothing friction and the air. Our ancestors made contact with the earth every day; it seems like a good idea to me.

Finally, spend time doing things that you love and laugh every day, even if it is at yourself.

In a 1990 interview, renowned chef Julia Child said, "Everybody is overreacting. If fear of food continues, it will be the death of gastronomy in the United States. Fortunately, the French don't suffer from the same hysteria we do. We should enjoy food and have fun. It is one of the simplest and nicest pleasures in life."

Food is what brings us together. Enjoy, and to your good health!

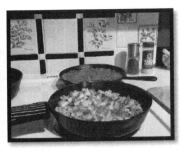

I usually cook without recipes or cookbooks—even though I collect them, especially old ones. For the first time I am attempting to write out a few of the favorites here at the Karr Homestead Kitchen.

I like simple food packed with health-promoting nutrition. It is the synergistic combination of the ingredients that yields energy and enjoyment while feeding your DNA with culturally appropriate nutrition. Remember that your cells carry the memories of your ancestors. They liked real food.

Berry Vinaigrette Salad Dressing or Glaze
1 cup mixed berries
1 cup balsamic vinegar
¼ cup raw honey, real maple syrup or stevia to taste
½ cup filtered water
½ cup organic extra virgin olive oil
¼ tsp turmeric, pinch black pepper

Place all ingredients into a blender and mix until smooth. Place dressing into a glass jar and refrigerate. This mixture is good for two to three weeks. Use as a salad dressing or as a glaze for salmon, cauliflower, broccoli or chicken.

Quinoa salad
2 cups cooked quinoa
2 chopped Roma tomatoes
2 cloves fresh garlic, chopped
1 bulb fresh fennel, chopped
1 bunch watercress, chopped
2 sweet red, orange or yellow peppers, chopped
1 medium yellow onion, chopped
2 medium green chilies, chopped
½ cup pine nuts or pecans
1 small bottle (12 to 16 oz.) creamy Italian salad dressing
OR
Mix together to taste:
Olive oil, rice vinegar, Celtic sea salt, black pepper, crushed garlic, turmeric, basil and dash of cayenne.

Mix everything together and eat fresh, warm or cold. Keeps well refrigerated.

Alaskan Summer
2-4 Alaskan salmon or halibut steaks

Place fish steaks on individual heavy aluminum foil sections. Top each steak with slices of summer squash, fresh tomatoes, sweet onion, fresh basil, chopped garlic and 1 tbsp. extra virgin olive oil.

Wrap tightly and place on grill at low heat (300 degrees). If the fish is thawed, cooking time will be about 15 minutes; 25 minutes if frozen or pieces are thick. When fish flakes but is still moist it is ready to serve.

Wild Rice Salad
Apple cider vinaigrette
6 Tbsp apple cider vinegar
1/4 cup wild honey
3/4 cup extra virgin olive oil, or clarified organic butter (melted)
Celtic Sea Salt and fresh ground pepper

Combine all ingredients, whisk or blend and let rest for 1 hour or up to 10 days refrigerated.

Salad
6 cups homemade vegetable stock or Pacific® brand
1 1/2 cups wild rice
1 carrot, peeled and cut into 2-inch matchsticks
3 Tbsp dried cranberries
1 plum (Roma) tomato, finely diced
4-5 scallions (green onions), including green tops, finely chopped
1/2 cup pine nuts, toasted and cooled
1/4 cup raw pumpkin seeds, toasted and cooled
3 bunches washed watercress stemmed

Combine stock and wild rice. Bring to a boil, and then reduce the heat to simmer. Cover and cook until tender (45 to 55 min). Spread the rice on a baking sheet and let cool.

Scrape the rice into a large bowl and add the carrot, cranberries, tomato, scallions, pine nuts and pumpkin seeds. Toss to mix.

Add 1/2 cup vinaigrette and toss and coat. Cover and refrigerate for at least 1 hour.

Divide the watercress among salad plates and top with the wild rice.

This adapted recipe comes from the traditional Ojibwa of the North American Great Lakes.

Taste of Italy
2 flank steaks (beef, elk or buffalo); Tenderize with the meat hammer, rub with extra virgin olive oil
1-2 cloves fresh garlic, chopped and sprinkled on each steak
2-4 asparagus spears

Slice summer squash, tomatoes, fresh basil and sweet onions. Spread veggies on steak. Add a pinch of black pepper and roll each steak with veggies in the middle. Use toothpicks or string to tie rolls and hold them together. Place in a glass baking dish, cover top of rolls with tomato sauce and a dash of Italian seasoning. Cover with foil. Bake at 350 degrees for 35 minutes. Serve with pasta.

Going Greek
½ lb ground lamb; form into small meatballs
2 red chili peppers, thin sliced
½ bunch fresh basil, chopped
4 pre-cooked red potatoes sliced into small pieces
3 cloves garlic, chopped or minced
1tbsp. extra virgin olive oil
Fresh ground black pepper
Celtic sea salt

In cast iron skillet warm oil; add chilies and garlic, then basil. Sauté for 5 minutes on medium heat and add lamb; brown the lamb then add potatoes. Cover for 10 minutes, add ground pepper and stir until mixed in. Cook for 5 minutes more. Salt to taste and serve.

Poultry Stock

While making stock is time-consuming, it isn't hard and it is well worth doing. Once you get used to having this versatile staple in your refrigerator, freezer or canned in glass jars, you will wonder how you ever got by without it. This versatile stock can be used almost anywhere stock is required. Using just bones is fine, but many birds' bones are hollow. To make up for this lack of marrow, meaty pieces like wings, backs and necks are usually added to poultry stock. You can mix and match the bones of different birds. The finished stock is the foundation for hundreds of soups.

Makes 7-8 cups

4 lbs poultry bones and backs, cut into 2- to 3-inch pieces (or any other kind of marrow bone)
2 medium carrots or yams, sliced
2 celery or lovage stalks, sliced
1 yellow onion, unpeeled, cut into wedges
2 leeks or scallions, trimmed and quartered lengthwise
6 flat-leaf parsley or watercress stems
3-4 mashed garlic cloves
1 large thyme sprig
1 large sprig rosemary
1 bay leaf
¼ tsp ground turmeric
¼ tsp black peppercorns
Celtic sea salt, to taste

1. Rinse the bones and backs under cold running water, then place in a large stockpot, along with the herbs and vegetables. Pour in enough cold water to cover the bones, about 12 cups, and bring slowly to a boil. As soon as the stock begins to boil, reduce the heat so that it simmers. Using a soup ladle, skim off any scum that has risen to the surface (rotate the bowl of the ladle on the surface of the stock to make ripples; this will carry the scum to the edges of the pot, and you can then use the ladle to lift it off). Add turmeric and peppercorns and simmer uncovered for 5 hours, skimming from time to time.

2. Strain the stock through a sieve into a large bowl. Discard the debris left in the sieve and cool the stock quickly by placing the bowl in a larger bowl or sink filled with ice water; occasionally stir as it cools. If you will not be reducing the stock, add about 1 teaspoon salt.

3. Refrigerate the stock for 6 hours or overnight to allow the fat to rise to the top and the debris to sink to the bottom. Remove the fat before using (and discard the debris at the bottom of the bowl). Divide into 1 cup quantities and refrigerate for up to 3 days or freeze for up to 6 months.

Italian White Bean Soup

1 Tbsp organic extra virgin olive oil
1 clove garlic, minced
1/4 cup onion, diced
1- 30 oz can white kidney beans or Great Northern Beans (do not drain)
1 1/2 cups water
1 1/2 tsp dried sage
1/4 cup celery seed
1/4 cup carrots, diced
1/2 cup fresh spinach, chopped or frozen
1/8 tsp ground black pepper
Celtic sea salt

Sauté vegetables in oil with herbs. Add beans, water and pepper to vegetables. Bring to boil and cook for 20 minutes. Reduce heat, add spinach and simmer for 5 minutes. Total cooking time about 25 minutes. Salt to taste after cooking.

Makes 4-5 servings.

Best Ever Broccoli Soup

4 cups chopped fresh organic broccoli (should be in 3-inch size to fit in the food processor)
3 cups fresh water
3 tsp Celtic sea salt
Fresh ground black pepper
Extra virgin olive oil
Place water, salt and broccoli in 4-quart sauce or stock pan. Bring up to a moderate boil stirring broccoli until tender and bright green.

Place broccoli with broth from the pan in the food processor—you may have to do in batches to not overload your processor. Process on puree until smooth—make sure you add enough liquid from pot to make a medium-thick soup. Place in bowls, top with ground pepper and a few drops of oil—serve hot.

Makes 3-4 servings

White Beans with Olive Oil & Parsley

1 30 oz can white beans, lightly drained
2 1/2 Tbsp extra virgin olive oil
1/8 tsp ground black pepper
1 1/2 Tbsp fresh lemon juice
3 Tbsp fresh parsley, chopped
1/4 cup red onion, minced

2-3 cloves garlic, crushed
Celtic sea salt

Place beans, oil, salt and pepper in a saucepan. Bring to a gentle boil. Reduce the heat to low. Add lemon juice, onion, parsley and garlic. Stir and serve hot. Salt to taste.

Yam and Ham Soup
3 medium yams, chopped into chunks
3-4 cloves garlic, minced
½ cup chopped shallots
½ cup chopped celery with green leafy tops
1 cup uncured ham chopped
1 stick organic butter
2 quarts Pacific® Organic Chicken Broth
1 can Thai Kitchen® Organic Coconut Milk

Place all the ingredients into a crock-pot or VitaClay rice/soup cooker on ready to eat setting. Or cook in a conventional stockpot, bring to a slow boil, cover and turn on low heat. Stir and serve with warm sourdough bread or gluten-free bread and organic butter. Warms up well and freezes also. Takes approximately 45 minutes.

Italian Salad Dressing
1/4 cup extra virgin olive oil
1/2 cup water
4 Tbsp balsamic or rice vinegar
2 Tbsp maple syrup
1 tsp dried basil
1/2 tsp dried oregano
3 cloves garlic, minced
1/4 tsp ground black pepper
1/2 tsp Celtic sea salt

Blend well in blender. Serves 8; Prep time about 5 minutes.

By the Sea
1 lb Mexican shrimp or prawns (scallops or chicken can be substituted)
4 Tbsp organic butter
4 Tbsp extra virgin olive oil
3 cloves garlic, minced
½ bunch fresh parsley, chopped
½ cup organic cream

¼ cup grated parmesan cheese
Fresh ground black pepper
Pinch Celtic sea salt (at table)

Add butter and oil to skillet, warm, add garlic and parsley, stir/toss for 5 minutes on medium heat; don't smoke your oil.

Add shrimp or scallops and cream. Cook until shrimp are pink but still tender (about 8 minutes). Serve over gluten-free pasta. Top with cheese and black pepper and garnish with chopped tomato.

South of the Border
4 boneless skinless chicken breasts
16 oz jar of El Pinto® all-natural hot green or red chili sauce
2 Tbsp extra virgin olive oil

Warm olive oil and place chicken breasts (can be frozen) in a skillet. Cover and cook on medium heat for 10 minutes. Pour chili sauce over the top of chicken and cover. Let slow cook for 30 minutes; chicken should be cooked through.

Shred the chicken into remaining sauce and use for tacos, salsa salad or sliced chicken and serve on a bed of brown rice or quinoa with beans and blue corn chips.

Pork & Fennel
4 organic pork loin steaks trimmed of fat
1/4 cup fresh fennel top, finely chopped
1/4 cup sweet onion, thinly sliced
1/4 cup fresh sweet basil, chopped
2 Tbsp extra virgin olive oil

Warm oil in a cast iron skillet. Lightly brown pork loin and cover with the rest of the ingredients. Cover with a lid and cook on medium-low heat until pork is done. Do not overcook the pork. Serve with rice, pasta or sweet potatoes and sliced apples.

Shrimp & Broccoli
15-20 medium prawns, peeled and deveined
2 cloves garlic, minced
2 Tbsp organic butter
2 Tbsp extra virgin olive oil
2 broccoli spears, whole or tops

Warm butter and oil in skillet, add garlic and shrimp. Toss over medium heat until shrimp turns bright salmon color. Cover with broccoli and then cover with lid for 5 to 10 minutes on medium-low heat until broccoli turns a bright green. Toss together and place on plates as is or serve with rice pasta topped with a sprinkle of parmesan cheese. Prep time 15-20 minutes, cook time 15-20 minutes; total time 35-40 minutes.

Roasted Cauliflower with Pomegranate Glaze
1 head cauliflower
Combine 1 cup pomegranate juice with
1/8 tsp turmeric
1/8 cup raw honey
2 cloves garlic, chopped
Fresh basil leaves to taste

Wrap in foil and bake on the grill or in the oven (325 degrees) until tender.

Ready in a flash one-pan dishes
Lightly steam broccoli with red onions, mild chili peppers (seeded) and Roma tomatoes. Top with a dash of Parmesan cheese and a handful of pine nuts.

Cook time 10 minutes or until tender—don't overcook.
Use amounts suitable for your family; it doesn't matter if you need 1 floweret, or ten.

Chop 1-2 bunches rainbow Swiss chard and add to warm skillet with 1 Tbsp. olive oil. Add chopped pecans, toss with chopped nuts until wilted, add ¼ cup balsamic vinegar, toss and remove from heat. Cook time is less than 10 minutes.

Sautéed Broccoli and Fresh Basil
4 cup broccoli flowerets
1/2 cup fresh basil
2 cloves garlic, chopped
2 Tbsp organic butter

In a cast iron skillet, gently melt the butter (lower heat to not burn). Add fresh basil and garlic; let basil wilt, add broccoli and cook on medium heat, tossing until broccoli is tender but not overdone.

Asparagus and Toasted Red Peppers and Garlic
1 bunch fresh asparagus
1 red pepper
1 cup fresh broccoli tops
2 cloves garlic
¼ tsp red pepper flakes
1 Tbsp extra virgin olive oil
1 fresh lemon

Wash and trim asparagus, using the top 4-5 inches that are tender. Wash and clean seeds out of red pepper, trim broccoli to the tender stems and tops.

In a cast iron skillet warm oil over medium heat; add sliced garlic and pepper flakes. Let garlic toast and add vegetables. Toss vegetables with oil and garlic, cover with a lid, and allow to steam on med-low heat till vegetables are bright in color and tender but still crisp.

Transfer vegetables to a platter, squeeze fresh lemon juice over vegetables and sprinkle fresh course sea salt on top. Serve warm or cold.

Sausage and Wild Grains
1 lb. Hormel® Natural Choice Smoked or Adel's® apple sausage
1 red sweet pepper, chopped into chunks
1/2 sweet onion, chopped
2 cloves garlic, chopped
1 small zucchini or summer squash, thick slices
1 cup broccoli flowerets
2 cups cooked organic wild rice, quinoa blend (recommend the use of a rice cooker for this)
1 Tbsp extra virgin olive oil

In a cast iron skillet over medium heat add olive oil, garlic and meat, sauté until meat is heated through. Add remaining vegetables, stir into meat, cover with lid for 10 minutes or until broccoli changes color to a bright green. Cover with the pre-cooked grain, gently mix together and serve.

Pork Loin with Fruit
2 lean pork loin steaks: Brown both sides in a skillet with 1 Tbsp extra virgin olive oil on medium heat.

Drizzle 2-4 Tbsp zesty Italian dressing over each browned loin, cover for 10 minutes.

Remove lid, and cover both pork loins with 2 cups frozen or fresh berries including cherries, raspberries, Marion berries, and/or blackberries.

Cover and turn heat to low, let slow cook for 30 minutes. Remove the lid and turn heat back to medium-low and let liquid evaporate for another 15 minutes. Serve with salad, cauliflower or wild grains.

Sautéed Radishes with Butter and Parsley
1 large bunch of radishes, sliced
1 good hand full of radish seed pods from those that have bolted in your garden
2 Tbsp organic butter
1/4 cup fresh parsley, chopped
Salt

In a large skillet or sauté pan, melt the butter and add the radishes. Sauté over medium heat for about 5-7 minutes. You want the radishes to soften, but still stay a little firm. Add the parsley and stir. Salt to taste. Serve immediately.

Buttered Cabbage
Serves 6-8
1 lb fresh savory cabbage
2-4 Tbsp Kerrygold® Irish Butter
Salt & pepper

Remove all the tough outer leaves of the cabbage. Cut head into fourths; remove stalks from center, then cut each quarter across the grain into fine shreds.

Put 2-3 Tbsp water into your cast iron pan together with butter and a pinch of Celtic sea salt. Bring to a boil, add cabbage and toss over medium heat, then cover and cook for a few minutes (don't overcook; this only takes 1-2 minutes). Toss again, add a pinch more salt and fresh ground pepper and top with a knob of butter (1Tbsp) and enjoy.

For those with more time: Sauté 1/2 cup thinly sliced yellow onion in warm butter just before adding the cabbage. Eat alone or with steamed red potatoes and Irish bangers (sausages).

I like to visit The Wellsprings School of Healing Arts in Portland, Oregon, to talk with holistic nutrition students. The class of 2015 introduced me to several new recipes; I have included two of them here. I hope you enjoy them as much as we do.

Thai Lettuce Wraps
By Tania Hunter Noel

Recipe may be doubled. May be made a day or two ahead of time; this allows the flavors to intensify.

Sauce Ingredients
1/4 cup raw wild honey, or agave
1/8 cup Nama Shoyu, or Tamari
1/2 tsp fresh garlic, minced
1 tsp fresh ginger, grated
1Tbsp hulled sesame seeds
1 Tbsp sesame oil

Filling Ingredients
1 1/2 cups raw walnuts
1/2 cup diced carrots
1/2 cup fresh cilantro, minced
1/4 cup scallions, minced (greens only)

Extra Ingredients
1 head lettuce, butter, bib, or romaine, leaves washed and dried
1/4 cup grated carrot

Directions
Prepare the sauce by adding all ingredients to a food processor and pulsing 3 or 4 times. Add walnuts and pulse an additional 4 or 5 times, until the mixture resembles ground meat. Add the carrots, cilantro and scallions, and continue to pulse another 3 or 4 times until combined. Place lettuce leaves on a plate, scoop 1 or 2 tablespoons of walnut mixture into center. Garnish with grated carrot.

Prep time: 15 - 20 minutes. Serves 10-12.

Coconut Date Rolls
By Vaughn Kimmons

Ingredients
1 cup of raw almonds, soaked (prior to beginning recipe, soak almonds overnight)
¼ tsp of sea salt
1 cup of pitted Medjool dates (about 10-12 dates)
A pinch of cinnamon (optional)
1 tsp of vanilla extract (optional)
1 cup of shredded coconut
¼ cup of roasted cashews for topping (any nut will be a great addition)

Directions
Place almonds and salt in food processor and process until the nuts are coarsely chopped. Next add the dates, cinnamon and vanilla and process until the mixture is thoroughly combined or begins to form a gooey ball-like shape. Then lay out a sheet of wax paper and evenly spread the coconut on top. With your hands, begin to form the date mixture into small cylinders.

For the finishing touches, roll the cylinders in the coconut until they are evenly covered. Place date rolls on a plate and gently press one cashew on the top of each roll. Goes well with mint tea. Store in an airtight container. Preparation time: 15 minutes.

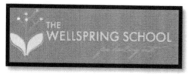

The Wellspring School of Healing Arts Portland Oregon - info@thewellspring.org

---

Trail Mix in Minutes
Use one bag each of the following from Costco® or a bulk food store; it costs a fraction of the prepackaged store brands, and there are no processed fats or added sugars.

Raw almonds
Raw pecans
Young Philippine coconut chunks
Dried cherries
Dried blueberries
½ bag dried cranberries
1 small bag organic dark chocolate chips

Combine all ingredients in a large 16-quart mixing bowl or container. Blend thoroughly with a spoon or your hands. Fill quart freezer bags, place in freezer, grab and go! Approximately 8-quarts.

Granola, gluten-free
1-2 lbs bag Gluten-Free Old-fashioned Oats from Bob's Red Mill®
1 cup dried cranberries or blueberries
1 cup chopped raw pecans
1 cup chopped raw almonds
1 cup Bob's Red Mill® coconut flakes
1 cup melted organic butter
½ cup warm local honey
1 tsp ground cinnamon
¼ tsp ground clove
1 tsp real vanilla

Mix dry ingredients with spices, breaking up any clumps of dried fruits. Add melted butter and warm honey, mixing well to distribute honey and butter evenly through mix. Heat oven to 300 degrees.

Place raw granola on jelly roll pan(s); spread out evenly and not too thick, place in oven for 15 minutes, stir to prevent burning or over-toasting on bottom and edges, cook for additional 15 minutes, stir once more. If edges are brown and the mixture has a nice golden brown color set out to cool.

Cooking times vary on local ingredients and elevation. Approximant cook time: 30 minutes. When cool place in glass mason jars with lids and store in fridge or freezer to preserve oil freshness.

Coconut Milk Ice-Cream
To make this you need an ice-cream maker. I like the Rival® 1 quart maker where you freeze the bowl, no messing with ice and salt; it's just the right size for 2-4 servings. Ready in 20-30 minutes.

1 can organic coconut milk
1/8-1/4 cup raw honey or real maple syrup
1/16 tsp xanthan gum (optional)
1 tsp real vanilla

Blend in a food processor, blender or by hand until smooth. Add flavorings listed below. Stir in chunk flavorings before placing in ice-cream freezer bowl. Follow mixer recommendations for freeze and set time. Enjoy!

Optional flavors:
- 1/4 cup dark cocoa powder with a pinch each of cayenne, cinnamon and ginger
- ¼ cup mixed frozen berries
- ¼ cup chopped nuts

- ¼ cup dark chocolate chunks

Blackberries & Peaches
Use a 9x13 inch glass baking dish
6-8 peaches, sliced (more if you like)
4 cups blackberries (more if berries are small)
Place fruit in the bottom of the pan.

Crumb Topping:
1 cup almond flour
1 cup brown sugar
½ cup organic butter
1 cup gluten-free rolled oats

In stand mixer, combine ingredients and mix well until butter is well incorporated. Spread topping over fruit. Bake for 35- 45 minutes at 350 degrees. Times will vary based on thickness of fruit, oven variances and elevation.

Baked Apples with Blackberries
2-4 tart apples, cored
1/4 cup blackberries
4 Tbsp organic butter
5 Tbsp organic brown sugar
1/4 cup water

Place apples so they do not touch in the pan. Fill centers with brown sugar and blackberries. Top each apple with a pat of butter. Cover pan with a tight-fitting lid.

Bake in oven at 350 degrees for 45 minutes -1 hour, depending on the size of apples.

Spiced Cider
1 quart apple or pear juice
1/2 tsp organic ground cinnamon
1/8 tsp organic ground cloves or allspice

Add juice and spices to the saucepan. Bring the mixture to boil then turn off and let cool. Serve warm or cold. You can also add cranberry juice or sliced orange without the peel to cup. Note: If you use whole spices be sure to remove them after juice cools or it will taste bitter over time.

Mexican Coffee
Brew up your preferred organic coffee and add the following to suit your taste:

2 Tbsp French vanilla coconut coffee creamer
Sprinkle of cinnamon
Sprinkle of cayenne pepper
1 tsp heaped organic cocoa powder

Place in bottom of the cup, add a little coffee to blend ingredients then finish filling your cup. Add organic sugar if you must.

Food of the Gods Chocolate Mousse
1 cup organic sugar
¾ cup organic butter
¼ cup organic cocoa powder
1 tsp Mexican vanilla
½ tsp cinnamon
1 oz Mexican tequila
Small pinch cayenne pepper
3 organic large eggs

Soften and cream butter and slowly add sugar, cocoa and spices, and then tequila and vanilla. Mix on med-high speed till well-blended. One at a time while mixer is running, add raw eggs (with a pause of 60 sec between each one). Turn the mixer to high and beat for a smooth froth (about 2 minutes).

Place a small amount into small dishes and place in the fridge to firm up (about 30 minutes). Serve with a topping of fresh organic whipped cream and a sliver of organic dark chocolate. This is very decadent and rich; it melts like silk in the mouth and will make chocolate lovers sigh.

Special thanks to the following historical groups and locations:

Bowman Museum—Prineville, Oregon
Heritage Museum— Independence, Oregon
The Deschutes Museum—Bend, Oregon
High Desert Museum—Bend, Oregon
National Archives —Washington, D.C.
National Food Exhibit —Smithsonian Museum of American History, Washington, D.C.
Old Town Historic District—Butte, Montana
Oregon Historical Society—Portland, Oregon
Portland Art Museum —Portland, Oregon

Oregon State Parks Service
Baker Heritage Museum—Baker City, Oregon
Frenchglen Hotel State Heritage Site—Frenchglen, Oregon
Kam Wah Chung & Co. Museum—John Day, Oregon
Pete French Round Barn—New Princeton, Oregon
Shore Acres State Park—Coos Bay, Oregon
Willamette Mission State Park—Salem, Oregon
The towns of Antelope, Drewsey, and Shanako, Oregon
The Whitman Mission—Walla Walla, Washington

National Parks Service
Fort Vancouver National Historic Site
McLoughlin House—Oregon City, Oregon

Special thanks to the following organizations and schools:

American Association of Integrative Medicine (AAIM)
National Association of Nutrition Professionals (NANP)
American Naturopathic Certification Board (ANCB)
The Wellsprings School of Healing Arts, Portland, Oregon

Special Thanks to My Mentors and Medical Advisor Team

Lorrie Amitrano, FNP-C, AHN-BC, CNP

Susan Barendregt, NT

Larry Boggart, MD, PhD

Darryl George, DO

Mary L. Hagood, FNP-C

Marty Hiers, RPh

Melissa McLean-Jory

Liz Lipski, PhD, CCN

Tom O'Bryan, DC

Jim Paoletti, FAARFM, FIACP

Kurt V. Rethwell, DC

Paul C. Robbins, LAc

Susan Tyler, CNC

James L. Wilson, ND, DC, PhD

David Zava, PhD

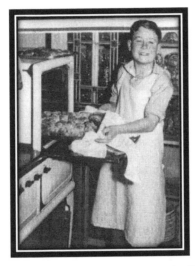

James Hare, 10 dimistrates his skills at Camp-Cooking Club of
4-H 1932, Portland Oregon OHS Image bb010773

Bibliography

Agriculture, U. S. (1935). *Yearbook of Agriculture 1935.* Washington DC: United States Printing Office.

Agriculture, U. S. (1942). *Keeping Livestock Healthy.* Washington D.C.: US Government Printing Office.

Agriculture, U. S. (1947). *Science in Farming.* Washington DC: US Government Printing Office.

Agriculture, U. S. (1951). *Crops in Peace and War.* Washington DC: United States Government Printing Office.

Alan Keith Tillotson, P. A. (2001). *The One Earth Herbal Sourcebook.* New York: Twin Streams.

Allport, S. (2006). *The Queen of Fats.* Berkeley: University of California Press.

Anderson, F. J. (1999). *An Illustrated History of the Herbals.* IUniverse Inc.

Balch, CNC, P. A. (2002). *Prescription for Herbal Healing.* New York: Avery.

Balch, CNC, P. A. (2002). *Prescription for Nutritional Healing the A-Z Guide to Supplements.* NY: Penguin Putnam Inc.

Barnard, N. (2013). *Power foods for the Brain.* New york: Hachette books.

Bellis, M. (2011). *History of Vitamins.* Retrieved from http://inventors.about.com/library/inventors/bl_vitamins.htm

Bland, J. (2014). *The Disease Delusion.* Harper Collins Publishing.

Blaylock, M. R. (1997). *Excitotoxins the taste that kills.* Santa Fe: Health Press.

Blaylock, M. R. (2006). *Sweet Deception.* Nashville TN: Thomas Nelson Inc.

Blaylock, M. R. (2009). *Aspartame, MSG and Excitotoxins.* Arizona: Truth Publishing International, Ltd.

Braly, M. J. (2002). *Dangerous Grains.* New York, New York: Penguin Putnam Inc.

Brown, P. S. (2000). *Better Bones, Better Body.* Los Angeles, CA: Keats publishing.

Brownstein, M. D. (2006). *Iodine - Why You Need It.* West Bloom, MI: Medical Alternative Press.

Brownstein, M. D. (2006). *Salt your way to health.* Westbrook, MI: Medical Alternative Press.

Buettner, D. (2008). *Blue Zones - Lessons for Living Longer From the People Who've Lived the Longest.* Washington, DC: National Geographic.

Calabrese C, M. S. (1999). A cross-over study of the effect of a single oral feeding of medium chain triglyceride oil vs. canola oil on post-ingestion plasma triglyceride levels in healthy men. *Alternative Medicine Review.*

Carter, J. S. (1996). *Vitamins.* Retrieved January 5, 2011, from http://biology.clc.uc.edu/courses/bio105/vitamin.htm

Centur, U. o. (2010). *Fish Oil Changes in Brain Cells via DTI Scan.* Dallas TX.

Chace, M. D. (1998). *What to eat if You Have Diabetes.* Chicago, IL: Contemporary Bokks.

Cichoke, D. A. (1994). *Enzymes & Enzyme Therapy.* New Caana CT: Keat's Publishing.

Civitello, L. (2011). *Cuisine and Culture: A history of Food and People.* Hoboken, NJ: John Wiley & Sons, Inc.

Cohen LA, T. D. (1998). The influence of dietary medium-chain triglycerides on rat mammary tumor development. *Lipids.*

Colbin, A. (1998). *Food and Our Bones.* Columbus, OH: Grade A Notes.

Collingham, L. (2012). *The Taste of War.* New York: Penguin Press.

Cordain, P. L. (2002). *The Paleo Diet.* Hoboken, New Jersy: John Wiley & Sons.

Cortes, M. (n.d.). *A Secret History of Coffee, Cocca & Cola.* Brooklyn: Akashic Books.

Cruess, W. (1948). *Commercial Fruit and Vegetable Products.* New York, Toronto, London: McGraw-Hill Book Company.

D.A. Lopez, M. R. (1994). *Enzymes - The Fountain of Life.* Munchen, Germany: Neville Press, Inc. .

Daniel, P. C. (2005). *The Whole Soy Story- the dark side of Americas favorite health food.* Washington, DC: New Trends Publishing, Inc.

Daoust, G. a. (2001). *The Formula - Personalized 40-30-30 Weightloss Program.* New York New York: Ballantine Books.

DicQie Fuller, P. D. (1998). *The Healing Power of Enzymes.* New York, New York: Forbes Custom Publishing.

Dow, J. (2012). *Beer from then to Now.* LuLu.com.

Doyle, M. D. (2008). *Nutrition for sports and exercise.* Belmont CA: Thomson Wadsworth.

Elson M. Haas, M. (2000). *The False Fat Diet.* New York: Ballantine Books.

Enig, P. M. ((2003). *Know Your Fats: The Compleat Primer for Understanding the Nutrition of Fats, Oils and Cholesterol.* Silver Springs MD: Bethesda Press.

Erasmus, U. (1997). *Fats that Heal Fats that Kill.* Burnaby BC Canada: Alive Books.

Fallon Sally & Mary Enig, P. (2001). *Nourishing Traditions.* Washington, DC: New Trends.

Fernandez-Armesto, F. (2002). *Near a Thousand Tables : A history of food.* New York, London: Free Press.

Fife, N. B. (2003). *The Healing Miracles of Coconut Oil.* Colorado Springs, CO: Piccadilly Books.

Fife, N. B. (2011). *Stop Alzheimer's Now!* Colorado Springs, CO: Piccadilly Books.

Foundation, T. C. (2010). *Fish Oil Effects on C-Reactive Protein Levels.* Cleaveland OH.

Gately, I. (2008). *Drink : A Cultural History of Alcohol.* New York: Gotham Books.

Gedgaudas, C. C. (2009). *Primal Body - Primal Mind.* Portland, OR: Primal Body- Primal Mind Publishing.

Germano, R. C. (1999). *The Osteoporosis Solution.* New York, New York: Kensington Books.

Gittleman, A. L. (2002). *Guide to the 40-30-30 Phenomenon.* NY: Contemporary Books.

Gladstar, R. (1993). *Herbal Healing for Women.* New York: Fireside Books.

Gladstar, R. (2008). *Herbal Recipes.* North Adams: Strorey Publishing.

Graveline, M. D. (2009). *The Statin Damage Crisis.* Duane Graveline, MD.

Green, M. P. (2006). *Celiac Disease - a hidden epidemic.* New York, New York: William Morrow.

Grieve, M. (1971). *A Modern Herbal Vol I & Vol II.* New York: Dover Publications.

Gruber, S. K. (2014). *The GMO Deception.* New York: Skyhorse Publishing.

Haas, M. E. (2006). *Staying Healthy with Nutrition.* Berkley CA: Celestial Arts.

Hetzler, R. (2010). *The Mitsitam Cafe Cookbook.* Washington Dc: Smithsonian National Museum of the American Indian.

Hewitt, J. R. (1872). *Coffee: Its History, Cultivation and Uses.* New York: Digital Text Publishing.

Hopkins, K. (2009). *99 Drams of Whiskey.* new York: St. Martin Press.

Howell, D. E. (1985). *Enzyme Nutrition - The Food Enzyme Concept.* Wayne NJ: Avery Publishing Group.

Hutchens, A. R. (1991). *Indian Herbalogy of North America.* Boston: Shabhala.

Ignarro, L. J. (2005). *NO More Heart Disease.* New York: St. martin Press.

In-Tele-Health. (n.d.). Hyperhealth - Encyclopedia of Nutrition and Natural Health. v8.0, www.hyperhealth.com, 360-626-8245.

Jensen, B. (1986). *Arthritis, Rheumatism, and Osteoporosis.* Escondido, CA: Grade A Notes Publishing.

Kamps, A. D. (2011). *What's Cooking Uncle Sam?* Washington DC: The Foundation for the National Archives.

Keal, B. (2008). *Tupperware Unsealed.* Gainsville FL: University Press.

Keane, M. M. (1996). *What to eat if You have Cancer.*

Keith, L. (2009). *The Vegetarian Myth.* Cresent City CA: FlashPoint Press.

Kirschmann and Nutrition Research, J. (2007). *Nutrition Almanac sixth edition.* NY: McGraw-Hill.

Kopec, N. D. (2013). *Let's Get Real About Eating.* Bloomington, IN: Balboa Press.

Kurlansky, M. (2009). *The Food of a Younger Land.* New York: Penguin Group.

Kurlansky, M. (2010). *Salt: A world History.* New York: Walker and Comp.

LaBella, L. (2012). *Seasoning CastIron.* Smashwords.

Lee, M. J. (1996). *What Your Doctor May Not Tell You About Menopause.* New York, New York: Warner Books.

Lee, M.D., J. R. (1999). *What Your Doctor May Not Tell You About Premenopause.* NY: Warner Books.

Legace, PhD, J. (2014). *The End of Pain.* Greystone Books.

Lemcke, G. (1906). *European and American Cuisine.* New York: D. Appleton and Company.

Lindlahr, V. H. (1942). *You Are What You Eat.* New York: National Nutrition Society.

Lipski, Ph.D, CCN, E. (2004). *Digestive Wellness.* New York: McGraw-Hill.

Loomis, J. D. (1999). *Enzymes - They Key to Health.* Madison WI: Grote Publishing.

Lowell, J. P. (2005). *The Gluten-Free Bible.* New york: Henry Holt and Comp.

Mabey, R. (1988). *The New Age Herbalist.* New York: A Fireside Book.

McK. Jefferies, M. F. (1996). *Safe Uses of Cortisol.* Springfield, IL: Charles C. Thomas.

Minger, D. (2013). *Death by Food Pyramide.* Malibu CA: Primal Blueprint Publishing.

Minich, P. C. (2009). *An A-Z Guide to Food Additives.* San Francisco, CA: Conari Press.

Montanari, M. (1949, 2004). *Food is Culture.* New York: Columbia University Press.

Mueller, T. (2012). *Extra Virginity: The Sublime and Scandalous World of Olive Oil.* New York, London: WW Norton & Comp.

Mulhall, M. J. (2008). *Saving Your Sex Life.* Munster, IL: Hilton Publishing.

Nathan S. Bryan PhD & Janet Zand, O. (2010). *The Nitric Oxide (NO) Solution.* Austin TX: Neogenis.

Nestle, M. (2006). *What to Eat.* New York: North Point Press.

Nestle, M. (2007). *Food and Politics - How the Food Industry Influences Nutrition and Health.* Berkley CA: University of California Press.

Nevin KG, R. T. (2004). Beneficial effects of virgin coconut oil on lipid parameters and in vitro LDL oxidation.

News, N. (n.d.). Retrieved 2010

Nieman, R. D. (2013). *Nutritional Assessment Sixth Ed.* New York: McGraw - Hill.

Northrup, M. C. (2001). *The Wisdom of Menopause.* New York, New York: Bantam Books.

NutraUSA.com. (2012, 11 26). Retrieved from http://www.nutraingredients-usa.com/Consumer-Trends/Huge-opportunities-in-the-emerging-cognitive-health-market-Enzymotec-USA-CEO

O., D. F. (2006). *The Beneficial Effects of Arctic Omega Liquid and ProOmega Liquid on Glucose Uptake and Cell Livability in L6 Muscle Cell Line.* Kingsville TX: Texas A&M.

O'Bryan, D. C. (Composer). (2006). Unlocking the Mystery of Wheat and Gluten Intolerance.

Orey, C. (2010). *The Healing Powers of Chocolate.* New York, New York: Kensington Books.

Peeke, M. M. (2000). *Fight Fat After Forty.* New York ,New York: Penguin.

Pendergrast, M. (2010). *Uncommon GFrounds: The History of Coffee and How it Transformed our World.* New York New York: Basic Books.

Pierce, T. (n.d.). *Outsmart Your Cancer.*

Pollan, M. (2001). *The Botany of Desire - Plants Eye View of the World.* New York New York: Random House.

Pollan, M. (2006). *The Omnivore's Dilemma.* New York New York: Penguin Books.

Pollan, M. (2008). *In Defense of Food - An Eaters Manifesto.* New York New York: Penguin Books.

Pottenger, J. M. (1983). *Pottenger's Cats - a Study in Nutrition.* Lemon Grove CA: Price - Pottenger Nutrition Foundation.

Quelus, A. L. (2011). *The Natural history of Chocolate.* Five Star Publishing.

Raawlings, N.D., Ph.D, D. (2008). *Foods that Helps Win the Battle Against Fibromyalgia.* Beverly MA: Fair Winds Press.

Reinagel, M. (2006). *The Inflammation Free Diet Plan.* New York, : A Lynn Sonberg Book.

Report, C. (July 2010). Protein Drinks.

Robinson, J. (2013). *Eating on the Wild Side - the Missing Link to Optimum Health.* New York: Bantam Books.

Ross, E. D. (2000). *Concepts in Biology Ninth Edition.* Delta College: McGraw-Hill Higher Education.

Rubin, J. (2010). *The Raw Truth.* West Palm Beach, FL: Garden of Life Inc.

Scheele, M. G. (2011). *The Obesity Cure.* San Diego CA: NovaLife.

Schuyler W. Lininger, J. D. (1999). *The Natural Pharmacy 2nd Edition.* New York: Random House.

Schwarzbein, M. D. (1999). *The Schwarzbein Principle.* Deerfield Beach FL: Health Communications Inc.

Schwarzbein, M. D. (2004). *The Program - losing weight the healthy way.* Deerfield FL: Health Communications Inc.

Sci., P. S. (2010). *Higher Intake of Omega-3 Fatty Acids Prevent an Excessive Response to an Inflammatory Stimulus.* University Park, PA: Penn State.

Shanahan, C. S. (2009). *Deep Nutrition - Why Your Genes Need Traditional Foods.* Lawai, HI: Big Box books.

Sharol Tilgner, N. (1999). *Herbal Medicine from the Heart of the Earth.* Creswell: Wise Acres Press.

Shawn Talbott, P. F. (2007). *The Cortisol Connection.* Alameda, CA: Hunter House.

Skidmore-Roth, L. (2006). *Mosby's Handbook of Herbs & Natural Supplements 3rd Edition.* St. Louis: Elsevier Mosby.

Smith, M. M. (2003). *HRT: The Answers.* Traverse City, MI: Healthy Living Books.

Smith, M. M. (2007). *Demystifying Weight Loss.* Traverse City, MI: Healthy Living Books.

Soram Khalsa, M. (2009). *The Vitamin D Revolution.* Carlsbad CA: Hay House Inc.

Staffan Lindeberg, M. P. (2010). *Food and Western Disease.* United Kingdom: Wiley - Blackwell.

Stephenson, M. K. (2004). *Awakening Athena.* Tyler, TX: Health, Heart and Mind Institute.

Stoll, M. A. (2001). *The Omega-3 Connection.* New York New York: Fireside Books.

T. Colin Campbell, P. (2013). *Whole - rethinking the science of nutrition.* Dallas TX: BenBella Books Inc.

Tabers. (2001). *Cyclopedic Medical Dictionary 20th Edition.* Philadelphia, PA: F.A. Davis Company.

Tannahill, R. (1988). *Food in History.* New York: Three Rivers Press.

Tason, M. (2011). *A Guide to History of Chocolate.* www.enjoyablebooks.com.

Thayer, P. R. (2001). *Calm Energy.* Oxford, NY: Oxford University Press.

Thornton, T. M. (2014). *Whole-Person Caring: An Interprofessional Modle for Healing and Wellness.* Sigma Theta Tau International.

Throop, P. (1998). *Hildegard von Bingen's Physica.* Rochester , VT, USA: Healing Arts Press.

Tilgner, N. S. (1999). *Herbal Formulas.* Creswell: Wise Acres Publishing.

Tribune, M. M. (2010). Meat Recall Affects Southern Oregon.

The University of California Dept. of Internal Medicine. (2010). *Fish Oil and Blood Flow in the Elderly.* Davis CA.

Wahls, P. T. (2014). *The Wahls Protocol.* New York, New York: Penguin Group LLC.

Watson, C. B. (2007). *The Fiber 35 Diet.* New York, New York: Free Press.

William Davis, M. (2013). *Wheat belly.* Rodale.

Wilson, B. (2012). *Consider the Fork.* Philadelphia: Perseus Books.

Wilson, N. D. (2007). *Adrenal Fatigue.* Petaluma, CCA: Smart Publications.

Winter, M. R. (1999). *Food Additives.* New York, New York: Three Rivers Press.

Wong, N. P. (2003). *Vitalzym - Total System Support.* Phoenix AZ: World Nutrition Inc.

Wright, M. J. (2000). *Vitality & Potency.* Petaluma, CA: Smart Publication.

Wrought Iron Range Co. (1925). *Home Comfort Cook Book.* St. Louis, MO.

Young, P. R. (2005). *The pH Miricle for Weight Loss.* New York, New York: Warner Books.

Tammera J. Karr, PhD, DAAIM, BCIH, BCHN, CGP, CNC, CNW, CNH, is an author, public speaker, educator and clinician. Tammera has served as the nutrition advisor to several wellness programs. She writes a weekly health column, reviews and contributes to national board exams, and is a contributor to online newsletters.

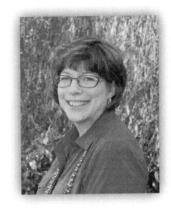

A native Oregonian, Tammera established an Integrative Medicine Partnership in 2006 and currently works in a clinical setting with DOs, FNP-Cs and others to provide clients with the tools needed to take control of their health. Her clinical and educational practice is always evolving to meet the needs of clients, the public and fellow practitioners striving to empower those they meet.